every day healing

every day healing

FINDING EXTRAORDINARY MOMENTS IN ORDINARY TIMES

ANN L. HALLSTEIN

THE PILGRIM PRESS   CLEVELAND, OHIO

To Nancy,
who has been alongside me down a
long and twisting path

AND

To my brother Robby,
who I wish were alive to read this

The Pilgrim Press, Cleveland, Ohio 44115
© 1999 by Ann L. Hallstein

Portions of several chapters appeared in vol. 2, no. 3; vol. 4, no. 1; and vol. 5, no. 3 of *The Living Pulpit* and are reprinted by permission.

Biblical quotations are from the New Revised Standard Version of the Bible, © 1989 by the Division of Christian Education of the National Council of Churches of Christ in the U.S.A., and are used by permission. May be adapted for inclusivity.

Printed in the United States of America on acid-free paper

04   03   02   01   00   99   5   4   3   2   1

Library of Congress Cataloging-in-Publication Data

Hallstein, Ann L. (Ann Lee), 1947–
    Every day healing : finding extraordinary moments in ordinary
times / Ann L. Hallstein.
        p. cm.
    ISBN 0-8298-1346-2 (pbk. : alk. paper)
    1. Healing—Religious aspects—Christianity.   2. Hallstein,
Ann L. (Ann Lee), 1947– .   I. Title.
BT732.H335   1999
234'.131—dc21   99-30794
                                                      CIP

contents

acknowledgments

I would like to convey my deep gratitude to all who helped along the way in the creation of this work, especially:

Each person I have written about here. You are modest, and being profiled in this way is not something you might choose. Your willingness to stretch your boundaries for the book is much appreciated, a gift.

Friends and loved ones who supported me along the way, believing in me when I needed it, including, first and foremost, Nancy Sykes and Chris Reese; Joey, Rini, Hal, Jay, and Hunk Hallstein; Thea Koehler; Lee Hancock; Judy Haigler and Connie Fender; Joyce Freeland; Amy Bruch; Edith Sullwold; Suzie Nakasian; and all others who gave encouragement, too numerous to mention.

Tony, for his prayers, which were indeed answered!

Smith College, for extending its libraries, especially Neilson, to the community for its use; the reference staff of Forbes Library, Northampton, Mass., especially Elise Feeley; and the Edwards Public Library, Southampton, Mass., for their able and willing assistance.

The *Living Pulpit*, a preaching journal, for its gracious permission to use passages of articles originally appearing in its pages, included here in "A Service of Healing," "Come into This Room," and "Trust Is Not Optional."

introduction

When I returned to my home in Massachusetts after six years in New York City, I realized that I was being healed of the harshness of the city and the intensity of life in a seminary simply by being here in a creative area filled with dedicated and talented people, surrounded by natural beauty, just *being* quietly in the world around me. I didn't know I needed healing, but I recognized it when it came my way because it felt so deeply nourishing, so enlivening. It then began to dawn on me that healing often comes quietly like this, through the still, small voice rather than through dramatic, miraculous ways. I believe in miracles, but I have learned that, though healing does indeed come in such ways, it tends to come oftener in more subtle, ordinary forms, so subtle that we might be inclined to miss these ways if we are not conscious of them.

This book was written so that anyone in need of healing will remember to look to his or her own life for agents of healing, to find in the ordinary course of daily life the extraordinary moments that can catalyze healing. Through my experience, I have discovered that healing opportunities are available right where we are. We don't have to go on a pilgrimage to find them. We tend to think that healing is something that happens "out there," somewhere else, to someone else, when it is right here, in this moment, awaiting us.

What do I mean by healing? Healing is a means by which a person comes closer to wholeness. Healing repairs what has been rent, restores what has been disenfranchised, empowers what has been disempowered, whether that is a body tissue or the soul. Healing is a way of concentrating what I call the life force to such a degree that it transforms something from an unhealthy state to a healthier one. It does not necessarily mean cure, though that happens too.

The life force is the energy or power that causes life to blossom, whether in a human or in a plant. It comes from God, the Source of all life. Believing that we were created by God to live and thrive and create and find meaning in life, I am convinced that God also equipped us with the means to do so, and that we have all we need to live healthy, whole lives embedded in the life around us, if we can just realize it. There are many modes of healing, many "agents," including people with certain talents, and all the many and varied manifestations of the creation that exist: beauty, music, nature, literature, quiet, architecture, laughter, and animals are some of these agents, and they can work on our behalf if we are open to their power.

The people in this book are real people I have encountered in my ordinary life. They carry some healing power by virtue of who they are and how they live out their lives. A few of them are in helping professions, but most of them wouldn't call themselves healers, and a few were shocked to learn I wanted to include them in this book! Nonetheless, healers they are indeed, because each has an attribute that is capable of contacting a person's soul with revitalizing force. And the soul must be tended if we are to live healthy and full lives. The medical establishment is finally beginning to learn that the state of the body reflects the state of the mind (because they are one functioning "unit"); the religious world has known for centuries that the soul must be "cured" for a person to live fully the life God gave.

"Curing" is a good word when used to mean the process that a soul goes through, over a lifetime, to grow into wholeness. A soul moves toward a state of health. A soul moves toward wholeness. A soul moves toward completion (not perfection). It takes time—in some cases a lifetime, in others less than that.

And in that process, in living out life as we do day by day by day, there are people (and other agents) who are a part of our daily lives with the capacity to move us along in the process if we are aware of them and willing to open ourselves to their power. That means seeing a person for who he or she truly is, being open to what we see, and being willing to receive what each one has to offer. Simple. Not easy, but simple. Healing is a mysterious, but not necessarily complicated, process.

It is my intention in sharing these life stories that you will consider and discover your own sources of healing. They surround you, even now. God does not leave you helpless. Look for what you need. It is there, waiting, provided by a munificent God.

a service of healing

A friend and I took off from work for a day trip to Baltimore one gray and misty Wednesday in the early eighties. We were both attending a course that surveyed a number of New Age topics, and the class was going on a field trip to the Mt. Washington United Methodist Church to see Olga Worrall, a famed healer. I was excited and a bit anxious, having never seen a healer before and not knowing what to expect. What if I was struck by some force and fell into the aisle? How embarrassed I would be! At that point in my life I still liked "things" to be under control (i.e., *I* needed to feel *I* was in control of myself and my environment), and a healing service seemed a place where "things" could very easily get out of control. (Much later I was to learn that healing is not subject to control, in that we never know when it may or may not happen, but this is very much a different thing from what I was worrying about on that particular day.) I had read about Mrs. Worrall, and I had seen pictures of her. In her photos she looked perfectly normal, kind, and grandmotherly: I recalled mature-looking dresses, maybe lace collars. That sense of her reassured me and kept my anxiety to a slight nagging, nothing unmanageable.

When we arrived at the church, in a modest working-class section of the city, buses jammed with people were starting to arrive. We parked and hurried inside to get a good seat. It was a standard-looking Protestant church, with a sizable congregation already in place. We found seats at the end of a pew and felt the charged energy of the atmosphere surrounding us. A sense of expectancy was in the air.

At the appointed time, three ministers processed forward from the back, including Olga Worrall. As they walked down the aisle, Olga was smiling, nodding, laughing, looking as if she was having the time of her life. Even though I'd seen her picture, I still had my own idea of how a healer would look. Olga definitely did not fit the role! She wasn't at all intense, and there was no Rasputin-like gaze in her eyes. She wore a plain black Geneva robe, the same as the other two, and her hair was pulled back into a somewhat loose bun. What I saw was an incredibly alive, very *present* person, somewhere in her sixties, the kind of person you might have had as a beloved second grade teacher or someone you were happy to bump into at the grocery store. She seemed enthusiastic, full of life, curious, kind, but not extraordinary other than the fact that she so appeared to be enjoying herself!

The other two were men, and all three took their places in the front. The senior minister of the church offered a few words of welcome and explanation about the service and how it was structured. It was to be a regular service with hymns and prayers, adding, of course, the opportunity to come forward for requests for healing and the laying on of hands. All three would do so; it wasn't just Olga "doing" the healing, and it was clear she was considered one of the ministers, not a star attraction, even though we were all there to see her. (I suspected everyone wanted to go to Olga, but by that time hundreds of people were crowded into the pews and standing in the back, and it was obvious we would be there all day if we all waited for her.)

We sang, we prayed, and finally we lined up for healing touch. Olga was still smiling, and while she listened carefully to each person and seemed to pray fervently, her eyes sparkled, her body was full of energy, and she maintained her enthusiastic demeanor. There was no whiff of piousness, no hint that she was anything other than humble. She was not someone wrapped in sanctity; she was just a woman being herself and doing what she had a talent for, opening herself to what heals and passing it along. I went to one of the other ministers, received his prayer and touch, did not fall out in the aisle (much to my relief!), returned to the pew, and started thinking about lunch. I was getting hungry, and we had plans to go to a tearoom in an old Maryland mansion for a crab lunch. I didn't feel "healed," and I wasn't transported into another world. I felt my stomach growling and was ready to go. At the time it seemed anticlimactic, and perhaps it was, for me. I had expected something more dramatic, people jumping up and throwing down crutches. The significance of what I witnessed didn't become clear to me until years later.

I did not realize then what I had participated in, and had no way of knowing that I had just learned one of the most essential aspects of healing, that it has to do with connecting to the life force. The life force, as I choose to call it, is the basic energy that creates and sustains life, and that emanates from God, the Source of life. Olga Worrall was in touch with that force, plugged in to the never-ceasing current that catalyzes life, that is life. Her laughter and enthusiasm came from her openness to life, which she let in with gusto. There didn't seem to be any defenses around her, nothing holding life outside the circumference of her being. She let it in, let it work in her and through her, and healing happened.

The life force heals on its own much of the time. When the body tissue repairs itself after a cut or when we spike a fever fighting flu, there is something at work in us doing the healing. Our bodies can heal themselves, but sometimes we need someone or something else to help heal us, an agent. The force for healing exists, and people are more or less skilled at perceiving it, opening to it, and using it (or more accurately, being used by it). The more sensitive one is to its existence, the more embracing of it, the more likely that person is to be able to mediate it to others. Olga Worrall was connected to it, it seems to me now, by the very fullness of her being, life attracting life. She clearly embraced life, and in her embrace she folded into herself its force, which she then shared with those who had less of it or a temporary loss of it. In this way was Olga Worrall a healer.

I had been disappointed when I didn't "see" any healings in the church in Baltimore because I didn't understand healing then, didn't know that it comes in ways that are hardly extraordinary, through ordinary people, albeit people with certain sensitivities. Certainly, there *are* the momentous events, the rare dramatic healings, the ones for which we may hunger. But much more common are the uneventful healings, the quiet ones, the ones that aren't noticed at the moment but are later obvious to us. The lesson I learned from Olga Worrall is that healing slips in through the mundane just as easily as through the awesome, and we may lose time, energy, and health looking for it in special places. Opening ourselves to the extraordinary in the ordinary, we open ourselves to the possibilities for healing that are present in every moment, all around us. Olga had a gift for healing, witnessed over the years by many other than myself, but she lived an ordinary life as a suburban Maryland homemaker. Healing is available in suburbs, from homemakers, from people who mow their lawns, line up at the post office, buy milk at the convenience store. We don't have to make a pilgrimage to Medjugorje or Lourdes. Healing is a possibility wherever we are (or a stone's throw away) if we are open to it as it presents itself. It may not happen just *because* we're open—after all, it's not under anyone's control—but being aware that the possibility exists brings it that much closer.

· 2 ·

digging potatoes

On a glorious morning one Sunday in October I sat in church gazing out the windows at the maple trees. Red was sparse that year. People thought it might be one more result of the summer's drought. Still, it was a quintessential New England fall day, with the huge old maples cutting through the bluest of skies and the light from the sun beginning to take on the golden hazy look that comes in those few select weeks before the faded white of the winter sun sets in.

On that particular Sunday I ached to be outside, stunned as I was with the beauty surrounding me on all sides. With the service finally over, I turned to the woman next to me, Kristina, and asked her if she needed any help digging up potatoes from her garden. I had seen her a week or two earlier, and she had mentioned that her niece had been over digging potatoes with her. It had sounded fun, especially when she mentioned getting the earth all over you as you sifted through it for the strays. It was a chance to get hands *and* body into earth. I have my own garden, but it's mainly perennials, with a smattering of vegetables. I had discovered when I came here many years ago from Washington, D.C., that there were plenty of people in the area from whom I could buy vegetables quite reasonably. That freed me to grow flowers, so there is a half acre of beds surrounding the house, including wild patches devoted to bees, butterflies, and hum-

5

mingbirds, of which there are plenty. But bringing in the harvest has a satisfaction all its own, and it was harvest time.

Kristina's mother, Peg, had just that week injured her leg, I was told, and that meant Kristina was doing double duty at home. They cook on a woodstove, keep Black Sex Link hens for eggs, and grow nearly all their own food. Their household is, as Kristina says, "labor intensive." My help would therefore be useful, but most of all I wanted to get to know Kristina better. I had met her that spring when we had worked together on a church restoration project, banding together to try to save our 250-year-old church from being vinyl-sided. Kristina and I and a few others worked together to gather information on the benefits of painting, Kristina doing the better portion of the work. The church did subsequently vote to repair and paint, including regilding the weathervane and four clock faces on the steeple. So all of this—church restoration and crisp autumn day and love of digging in the earth and Kristina herself—went into my offer of help, which was quickly accepted and set for that very afternoon.

Kristina was sorting onions in the garage when I arrived. She took up a pitchfork, and we headed out to the long row of potatoes. The method for digging potatoes with two people is that one person digs, as gently as possible so as not to spear into the potatoes, while the other sorts through the freshly dug portions to gather up the potatoes, brushing off the dirt before tossing them into a bushel basket. A little probing is necessary because smaller potatoes (called "pigs" because they are fed to pigs) may stay hidden underneath unless discovered by nimble fingers. Kristina had set out two kinds of potatoes that spring, red new potatoes and the rich yellowy Yukon Gold, recommended to her as a tasty good grower by the man at the feed store in Easthampton.

At our backs were a row or two of cornstalks, now dead but being saved to make the booth for Kristina's sister-in-law's Succoth celebration at her temple. The garden, a good-sized one, stretched back to a field that was itself backed by woods. Wild turkeys had come through the field recently: Kristina's neighbors, older and around the house much of the day, had called to report the sighting. The air was cool, but the sun warm, and there was an urgency to the gathering in, some anticipation in the air that stimulated our energy for work. The soil was rich and loamy and loose, pleasurable to finger through and not yet cooled by the waning of the sun. It was work of the earthiest, most primary kind, satisfying on a soul level, but also hard work, hard on the back, so that we took turns pitchforking and soon swung into a rhythm together, forking and digging. We talked, both of us content to be there.

A master furniture maker, Kristina makes pieces of pure and simple beauty that are often intricately carved with the techniques she learned from a Fijian woodcarver, Makete, when she was granted a Fulbright scholarship to go there to study with him. Like her work, Kristina is lean and tidy looking, all pure line, with precise, deliberate movements and speech. On this day she was open and centered, and it was obvious to me that she was in her place, at home in the most profound sense, her strong hands covered with earth and her trim body moving easily as she bent over the fork, digging. We worked like this for a few hours, loading three or four bushel baskets with potatoes, and then went in to have tea with her mother. I left laden with potatoes, fresh eggs, and bunches of just-ripened Concord grapes.

I boiled three of the red potatoes that night for my supper and had them along with a glass of red wine. I selected ones that had been speared and needed eating quickly, and they were the best I'd ever had, unlike any I had ever tasted. And as I sat eating those potatoes so redolent of the earth, tired in the good way that comes from physical labor, I realized that the afternoon had been a healing one, and that the healing came from being in the presence of one perfectly authentic person in one perfect place. We had been in sync, rhythmically entrained there in the sun and air and soil, Kristina totally present. Kristina's authenticity was somehow highlighted by the garden; it could be strongly sensed there and taken in. She had revealed her self there among the cornstalks, and a true self is whole and healing. Wholeness heals because nothing is to be added to it. Anyone being totally true to herself cannot help giving healing because she is giving of complete life. It was just by Kristina's presence that I was healed, and by that I mean I felt energy move around in my body and pervade me with a sense of well-being, with all being right with the world: I was made aware of my own wholeness. In that moment I was connected to Kristina, to all of nature, and to the creative Source of all being. Healing was done in the ripened garden and open field. A harvest was gathered in.

3
doctors dan

I know two doctors named Dan, both of them healers. The first Dr. Dan was a psychiatrist and family friend when I was growing up just outside Cleveland, Ohio. My parents played tennis every week, and one of the people they regularly played with was Dr. Daniel Badal, nicknamed by my father "Dr. Dan the Bandage Man." Dr. Badal was tall and lanky, with soft eyes and bushy eyebrows, and he smoked a pipe that he drew on slowly. His voice was wonderful: he conveyed an enormous amount simply by speaking—kindness, patience, interest—regardless of the words spoken. When he came over, either for dinner after tennis or for parties, he was the one adult I veered to immediately, for he treated children like people. He would crane his neck down, look me straight in the eyes, ask questions, and then really pay attention to whatever I said in response, never hurrying to get back to the adults, seeming to enjoy talking with me. Often he would steer me to a quiet corner so that we could talk without being interrupted. My main competition for his attention was my grandmother, Nana, who lived with us. Dr. Badal liked and appreciated Nana, who was an intelligent, well-read, erudite, and extremely kind and gentle woman. I loved her dearly and usually deferred to her in all matters, but I did try to make end runs around her in order to "get" to Dr. Badal first!

At ages eight, ten, twelve, I was shy, but I always drew near to Dr. Badal confidently, happy to deliver a drink or an appetizer, glad for any excuse to approach him, though none was needed, of course. As I look back, it seems that he sought

9

me out just as much as I sought him, but that may be a child's memory. I *do* know we connected, and the connection has lasted for years: I last saw him a year or two ago at my father's eightieth birthday party. Before that, I was a guest in his home after my mother had died; I was in town to disassemble my parents' house when my father moved to an apartment, and Dr. and Mrs. Badal invited me to stay with them, a godsend at the close of hard and emotional days sorting through my family's past. I have grown even more appreciative of Dr. Badal over the years, knowing now how few people really take the time to try to know children.

What Dr. Badal was doing for me during those encounters, I see now, was helping to give me a sense of self, helping me to grow into an individual who was more than the role assigned to me by my family. I didn't know what he saw in me at the time, but I did know he saw *something*, something that drew him to me. What mattered were his attention and his responding to me as an individual rather than as a child. By meeting me on equal footing, he added to my sense of personhood. I was a person worthy of his attention. I was more than a "mere" child: I had something to offer, to a psychiatrist at that! Esteemed in his profession, respected by my parents, Dr. Badal was someone with standing in the world, and yet there he was, standing with me. A child, or the child I was, doesn't always have words to describe what she feels, what she knows, but I knew on some deep level that Dr. Badal saw me for who I was. He saw who I was capable of growing into, my possibilities, and he respected me for it. He had insight, and he used it on my behalf, conveying quite clearly to me, "You are a special and interesting young person, and I am happy to know you," a message *every* child needs to get, as early as possible, as often as possible.

This message is, in fact, something every *human being* needs, regardless of age: to be treated with respect simply for being the person he or she is. Call it respect, call it compassion, call it love; whatever it is, it is the wonderful feeling that you are known, and who you are is just right. If we can accept ourselves as "right," just as we are, we are well on our way toward being the whole person that each of us was created to be. Not perfect, but whole. To see ourselves in such a way doesn't come easily for most, and it can require someone else seeing us as just right to persuade us. Seeing people as just right and conveying it to them was something Jesus did (certainly, he paid no attention to the conventional categories of "wrong" in his day) and was part of his healing abilities. Jesus is the more extreme example, but other, more ordinary people convey the same healing message, and Dr. Dan Badal was, and is, one such person. Drink in hand, puffing on his pipe, wearing white tennis shorts and a cable-knit V-necked sweater, he bore gifts of wholeness to a child yearning to know who she was—extraordinary moments in the suburbs of Cleveland, Ohio, in the fifties and sixties.

The other Dr. Dan I know is Daniel Smith, M.D., head of a department at Columbia-Presbyterian Medical Center, New York City. I first came to Dr. Dan in desperation, having been told by a rude and careless doctor in a horrid HMO that I had a tumor that could be cancerous. He wanted to operate, but would do so only if I signed a release that gave him carte blanche to remove anything he wanted from my body while he was "in there" because he didn't want to have to "mess around" and go "back in" a few weeks later, just so I could have time to make an informed decision about any condition he might discover. I wasn't about to sign over any parts of my body to his discretion. From what I had seen of him, he had none. The incident that sealed my decision was overhearing him tell an elder patient who was crying in his office, asking him what was going to happen to her, to stop worrying because we all have to die sometime. His caustic words astonished me. I walked out of his office right then, determined never to deal with him again.

I had just finished seminary, had no money, and so prayed for help, which came swiftly. I got the idea to call Columbia-Presbyterian, where I had been a chaplain, to try to find a good doctor and see what, if anything, could be worked out. I am absolutely certain that God herself guided me to Dr. Dan, because as soon as I entered his office, I knew I was safe, I knew I could trust him, and I knew I would be all right. This Dr. Dan has every reason to be arrogant. He heads a department in a prestigious medical center, has offices off Madison Avenue, possesses sterling credentials, lives in a posh suburb of New York City, is tall and attractive—the list continues, I'm sure, though I don't know more details. But I do know that he is far from arrogant. He is down-to-earth, warm, and not at all patronizing. Furthermore, he listens, pays attention, and cares about his patients. Lanky, friendly, with a wide smile and lively eyes, he is not aloof; he is entirely approachable.

Above all else, Dr. Dan is a healer in the best tradition, a physician who knows that there is much more to healing than technology and technique and training can afford. He is so unusual in this way that I once asked him where he thought his ability to heal, and his authority as a doctor, came from, and he responded immediately, "From God." He told me he knew that he had certain skills, and that he was the one responsible for bringing them to bear on a patient, but that all he was and had by way of talents and skills came from God. He felt an obligation to God to use his gifts effectively and carefully. He said he also knew that when a patient came to him with advanced cancer, although he might not be able to cure her, he was able to stand with her until the end, and that this "standing with" is part of his work as well (for one can be healed into death was what he meant, I presume). That "standing with" is not something many doctors seem capable of, and in Dan's case, I think it must come from his strong faith. A doctor calling on faith in going about the work of healing! It should not be extraordinary, but I'm sad to say it is. (I know that Dr. Dan acts on his faith in other ways too. An ordained elder in the Presbyterian Church U.S.A., he joined a team of doctors who volunteered at a medical clinic in Haiti, and he relished the experience.)

He may have shared this information with me because I am a minister—his patients would not necessarily know it, but they surely know the fruits of it, which is Dr. Dan's enormous capacity to inspire trust and hope. When one who is sick goes to a doctor, this is precisely what is needed to begin any healing: the feeling that the doctor can do something to make it better. More than anything he or she actually does by way of medicines dispensed, the doctor's attitudes and unspoken values will influence the patient. We know something about this from the placebo effect—that a patient given a dummy pill, delivered with authority and optimism on the part of the doctor, may improve. When the doctor's presence conveys compassion, respect, and caring, the patient senses that he or she will indeed be cared for, healed. This is Dr. Dan's gift: his confidence in his abilities, his love for his work and his patients, his sense that God is at work through him, all woven together to clearly signal to any patient, "You are safe with me, and you will be safe with me no matter what the outcome of your condition may be. I will be with you the entire way." Given such a message, who among us would not commence healing? I know I did, and the "healing medicine" Dr. Dan gives is so powerful that I make eight-hour round-trips to New York City to see him when another doctor would suffice. He is *not* any doctor, however. "Ordinary" man, extraordinary doctor, he is a healer, and that makes all the difference.

· 4 ·

life is change

Cynthia Sexton is an "intuitive counselor." That means she uses her intuition to help people understand themselves, the path they are on, the forces at work in their lives. In a one-and-a-half- to two-hour appointment Cynthia sits down with the client and proceeds to tell this individual everything that she intuits about him or her. The session is taped, so the client can go back to the information later. Sometimes she says things that make no sense at the time but years later, on relistening to the tape, become perfectly clear.

Cynthia doesn't make predictions about a person's life and doesn't consider herself a psychic. She has an extraordinary gift to see people, and she can "see" things that most of us cannot. What she does isn't that different from what most of us do when we get a first impression of someone that turns out, usually, to be quite accurate. First impressions are based on the multitude of data we gather, instantly, from someone we have just met. We are rarely aware of all that goes into forming the impression, but senses, experience, body types, and intuition all play a part in the mix. What Cynthia does seems much the same, different perhaps only in scope and depth. She is able to "get" more than most people do on a first meeting with you. She gets whatever comes to her and then feeds it back, information that helps you to see yourself through someone else's eyes, always with a caring, sensitive touch in terms of what you are told. Cynthia would never give any information that would lead to fear. She gives only data that can be helpful in looking at your life and trying to discern what needs discerning.

Once a nurse, Cynthia felt called into a new vocation and established a practice for herself in Maryland, currently in Chevy Chase. Her two careers are closely connected: she still cares for people, helps them heal, but no longer does it hands-on. Instead, she uses her gentle, caring way, her concern for your well-being, and her ability to know what ails you to help you do the work of healing yourself. She "touches" something inside you that sets off a reaction, and if you allow the reaction to blossom, it leads you somewhere that you need to go, helps you to do something you need to do in order to accomplish a change in life, moves you into a new place.

Change, in my experience, is rarely easy, even when it's something you want to do, and Cynthia is someone who points you to change, so sometimes her message is a difficult one to take in. Sometimes you hear things from her you would rather not. But as she reminds you, time and again, life *is* change, and to refuse change is to deny life. This might be Cynthia's theme, or certainly was her theme with me. Here is a change you are being confronted with. Will you accept it?

I remember the first time I went to see her. She knew nothing about me. I had come to her because I was considering change in job at the Library of Congress, where I then worked. I was a manager, but a restless one, exhausted by the bureaucracy and all its rules and regulations. Getting anything creative done took a massive amount of energy, time, and persistence. I was mulling over the idea of returning to my former work as a reference librarian, where I could do the work I liked, helping people find what they need, rather than live in the frustration I felt at trying to "manage" people in an unmanageable situation. Practically the first words out of

Cynthia's mouth were something to the effect that I needed to continue to develop the extroverted side of myself, that any situation in which I worked alone would not serve me. As an example, she said, it would not be good for me to work as a librarian! I needed to work as a manager in order to continue to develop skills that could come only by working with people. I was instantly deflated: her counsel was the precise opposite of what I wanted to hear, what I indeed had come for! She went on to give more detail, explaining why this seemed to be the case for me. It all made chillingly good sense, but it was not the direction I had picked for myself. To take it in, I would have to reorient myself. I would have to change.

Since that time I have learned, in working with people who come to me as a minister, that perhaps one of the most common reasons people get sick in body or soul is that a change needs to be made but they do not want to make it. I would say that this is a universal experience, or as close to universality as it comes (and I am one who uses the term sparingly). Change is hard for most people: it affects our wiring somehow. Even when we know we need to do it, whatever it is, it can be excruciatingly painful. It is often easier to deny it, put it off indefinitely, or plunge ourselves into other things, anything to take the focus off the change that is there, waiting for us. If we refuse it for too long, it works its way into our systems, causing all kinds of havoc, physical, psychological, spiritual. A loving person like Cynthia can heal, though, by pointing out what needs looking at, what needs doing. She has nothing invested; she is objective; she simply says what she sees. We can hear from her something we might not hear from someone close to us, who may more likely (and with reason) point out the way in which we need to change with editorial comment: why we should, how important it is, how not doing it is holding back the relationship, and so on. And as we know, that kind of counsel rarely helps us move forward. Rather, it may cause us to dig in our heels.

Cynthia is able to give you the benefit of all she can see about you, and she sees quite a bit. She sees who you are, what your gifts and talents are, and how they could be used effectively. She sees the issues you struggle with, the effects of your upbringing, the blocks that confront you.

She sees what is working for you in your life and what is not. And then, ever so gently, she suggests the changes that would help you move closer to where you need to go. To be given such help by someone with no agenda is healing. It heals because you need help, often, to bring something new into being, just as women need help to give birth to babies. You can do it alone, yes, but it surely is easier when you have someone with you! To hear from someone else, someone not "in" your life, what you need to know, what you must face if you are to grow, makes it less of a threat, more of a boon. It can make the change palatable. It can even make the change exciting!

The rhythms of life are just that, rhythms, and they need to move through us, and we must move in response to them. Stilling them, even briefly, can set up disharmony, and disharmony can make us ill. Attendant to rippling rhythms, midwife to change, Cynthia Sexton heals by seeing what needs doing and bringing it to our attention, using her extraordinary gifts on behalf of others, daily, in Chevy Chase, Maryland.

· 5 ·

the right place

Three places I know impart healing. In these three spots, setting and architecture combine to create places that draw in those who stop there and call out something that has the power to heal. Northampton, Hancock Shaker Village, and Seiji Ozawa Hall, Tanglewood, are the places, all within an hour of one another in our end of Massachusetts.

Northampton is a town of some twenty-nine thousand people set in the portion of the Connecticut River Valley between Springfield and Greenfield known as the Pioneer Valley (or more colloquially the Happy Valley). Voted the number one small town for the arts in America, it is home to Smith College, artists and artisans of all stripes, several coffee bars and ice cream parlors, and a variety of restaurants and shops that draw people, increasingly, from a wide circle around it. It is a place where people stroll up and down Main Street like promenading Italians, but here we stroll even in subzero weather, ice cream in hand. Teenagers play hackey sack and skateboard in the park, street performers gather knots of people on corners, children can play without fear, and lesbians (of whom there are many, earning Northampton the sobriquet Lesbianville, USA) feel free to be themselves. It is a colorful and mellow congregation of souls who gather here.

Coming into Northampton from the west, you see the hills of the Holyoke range that look like a stage setting for the center of town, especially on bright and sunny days when the mountains stand out against blue sky. There is a slight drop coming in from this direction and a moment at the stoplight just by the gates to Smith where you can take in the whole scene at a glance. It satisfies the spirit, that view. Then at the bottom of the incline, once level with the buildings, you are immediately aware of the scale: the scale of everything feels just right, from the classical Academy of Music (our movie house) on the corner to the parking garage, which blends unobtrusively and rather charmingly with its neighboring buildings. Main Street is angled in such a way that the brick buildings, mostly three to four stories and painted pale colors, seem to invite you toward them. The architecture makes me feel I am the "right" size, neither too big nor too small, for its scale fits my scale. In this place I feel right in body, mind, and spirit, empowered rather than diminished. It gives me a sense of agency and also of responsibility. I feel a part of the community, drawn in to something larger than myself. In my imagination, it seems as if this is how I'd feel were I part of a tribe somewhere, a village tribe. And I am not the only one who feels this way. It's a common experience, and though individuals might express it in different ways, what is sensed is palpable and shared.

I know little about architecture, but this architecture must be good, it seems to me, because isn't that how we *should* feel where we live, empowered? We know that slums oppress and depress, robbing people of vitality and initiative. Somehow Northampton lifts the human spirit and infuses it with vitality. It calls artists and writers and musicians and dancers here with that vitality; it breeds creativity. There is something that quickens the spirit in this place, and you take it in simply by being here. Vitality, empowerment, quickening: energy moving us more fully into life, healing, as does any greater connection with life.

Hancock Shaker Village is a restored Shaker community set in the Berkshire Mountains outside Pittsfield, on the far western border of the state. A dwelling house, meeting house, and round stone barn are there, along with smaller buildings for spinning and weaving, laundry, furniture making, blacksmithing, and the like. There is an herb and vegetable garden, and livestock are kept. The buildings are painted in distinctive colors—mustardy yellow, barn red, slate blue—and contain Shaker furniture and implements.

No "big money" seems to back this restoration, as the Rockefellers did Williamsburg; it's a more local effort, thus small scale, manageable, and rarely crowded. That, in fact, is part of its charm: there is no urgency to hurry through, no sense that it can't all be easily taken in. It doesn't feel like an institution. Though certainly a slice of American history and culture are experienced there, it is a place that can be apprehended through body and soul. Words are not necessary. The buildings speak for themselves.

Shakers worked hard from dawn to dusk, but work was a labor of the spirit as well as of body and mind, and spirit is nourished by the aesthetics of the design and construction. These buildings were clearly built to serve the human beings using them, built to make life more productive. Everything there—buildings, tools, furniture, clothing—functioned to serve life and to enhance, rather than diminish, the soul, unlike so many places where people have been required to work.

What I feel at Hancock comes directly from the place itself rather than from anything I know about the Shakers. There's something about the proportion and scale of the buildings, the purity of line, the richness of the woods in the floors and furniture, the positioning for light, the colors, all of this working together to make me feel that I "fit" there. The Shaker song "Simple Gifts" says,

'Tis the gift to come down where we ought to be.
And when we find ourselves in the place just right,
'Twill be in the valley of love and delight.

Shakers had an understanding of the power of being in the right place (both theologically and physically), and they worked to make their village right for those who lived there. What they knew, but what we have lost sight of in our society, is that our surroundings, our habitats and places of work and play, need to serve our humanity and spirit. We need to live where we can be reminded of the "rightness" of our humanness and feel connected to the earth and nature and God. We need proportion. We need harmony. We need "fit." When we live so, vitality increases because it is not being drained off by what is unnecessary or by what doesn't fit. At Hancock, the Shakers long gone, that vitality is available even now. To be physically in that place enlivens. It inspires. It quickens. It heals because there life is served and magnified.

Seiji Ozawa Hall is the newest concert hall at Tanglewood, the summer home of the Boston Symphony Orchestra, named after its music director. The hall opened in 1994 to great fanfare and reviews, some of which I remember reading. But I went to hear chamber music there only later, so had forgotten most of what I had read or heard. Thus, an utterly overwhelming surprise greeted me when I came down the path from the woods, emerging into the open space that surrounds this magnificent building.

Architect William Rawn of Boston designed the hall to fit into the once agriculturally based countryside that surrounds it. It has a barnlike look to the exterior, red brick with exposed wood beams and rafters, and huge natural-wood doors (in the process of weathering) at one end that open the hall to the people sitting on the lawn outside.

Inside, it is a fortuitous blending of classical lines interpreted with great originality to create a calm, almost Zenlike atmosphere. The ceiling soars, but is softened by its gentle arching. There are two balconies as well as orchestra seating; the balconies face five long, narrow windows at the other end, windows opening onto the trees and hills beyond. Behind the balcony seating are sliding doors that are opened during concerts, giving fresh air to even the seats farthest back. The walls are painted cream, the chairs are wood with forest green cushions, reminiscent of camp furniture, and there are red acoustical panels that line the rear of the stage. Taken all together, the feeling created is one of perfection: perfect setting, perfect proportion, perfect place.

Just sitting in this building is enough to make you feel washed with calm and peace, but when the music begins, it becomes a spiritual experience. The music, played by masterful musicians, is perfect, as are the acoustics. The calm quiet of the place comes alive with the music, which carries sparkling life into the space, the life force in action. The Brahms Quartet No. 3 in C Minor, played with purity of tone, of timing, of interpretation, made time drop away, carrying me to a place of pure proportionality. I knew, in this extraordinary moment, that there is at the heart of life a place of divine proportion of which music and architecture are reflective. Through music, we can "go there" in some fashion or at least sense it enough to take a sample of it into our being. Such purity of sound is healing because in that moment something in us is congruent with that perfection. We resonate with it, and it restores us to that "place" we so miss and long for. To hear music played in a place of such vision, a place that itself reflects the divine proportion, to be immersed in such pure beauty for even a few minutes, takes us to the very center of the Source of life, restoring us momentarily to wholeness, to the proportions each of us was born to know. For the price of a lawn ticket, an extraordinary moment of healing is there for the taking among the coolers and the blankets and the lawn chairs and people sprawled out, eating salads and tortes, sipping champagne, drinking in perfection.

It took me a while to realize that Northampton, Hancock Shaker Village, and Ozawa Hall have something in common: they are three places that somehow hold a capacity for healing. When I think of places for healing, I think of shrines, such as Lourdes with its waters or the holy wells of Ireland: natural places, that is, but not buildings themselves, not architecture. A book by Jonathan Hale called *The Old Way of Seeing* (Houghton Mifflin, 1994) gave me a possible explanation for what I have observed and experienced in these three places, however.

The Golden Section is a ratio used in construction to give true harmony of proportion. The ratio, which is 1:1.618, is such that if a straight line is divided into two parts, the ratio of the whole to the larger part is the same as the ratio of the larger part to the smaller. It was used in building the Great Pyramid of Cheops, the Parthenon, and Chartres Cathedral, and it has been known since the fourth century B.C.E. During the Renaissance it was called the divine proportion, which is fitting, because it is, as I understand it, the proportion that best fits us humans. "Proportion is the nature of architecture," says Hale. "There is an innately understood grammar of shape. And that grammar, unlike speech, is expressed in all living things. Euclidean shapes—cones, cubes, spheres—are often used to make architecture, but the deep patterns come from life forms." I take this to mean that the principle of proportionality is not just aesthetically pleasing, but somehow *in us,* an archetype residing in our psyches, perhaps, or coded in our DNA. The human body has numerous Golden Section proportions, according to Hale. Could we somehow be holographs of a universe of proportion? A universe whose elegant proportions add up to a great Wholeness? Our response to perfect proportion seems an expression of physical/psychological/spiritual *need*. That need (or longing) is for wholeness, reflecting the greater Wholeness, and the Golden Section is one mode through which we can "converse" with it: a grammar, to use Hale's word. When we are exposed to the Golden Section, we may be taking in a "dose" of wholeness, healing medicine for the body/mind/spirit.

The quickened feeling present in these three places may be the power of proportion at work. Right proportion, right shape, makes us feel more alive, and I believe it has the capacity to actually *make us* more alive. By engaging the life force and setting it into form, architecture both catalyzes and mends. Hale says it thus (italics are mine): "A great building, even a good building, does not merely create an effect of power, *it brings out our own power.* A building is not nature and it is not an imitation of nature; it is an expression of *our* nature."

Jonathan Hale comes at the concept of buildings being life giving through his work as an architect. I come at the same concept through my experience of place. What is important is that proportion and shapes, buildings and places, hold power for us, and yet are ordinary parts of our everyday lives. They present opportunities to discover places of healing right where we live. One room will do; one room to work on us, to evoke our own power, to call out the life that is always inside us until we die. When we find our way to a place of harmonious proportion, to the place just right, healing can happen.

· 6 ·

a hot tub meeting

I first met Edith Sullwold in a hot tub, outside, at night, so all I first knew of her was pure presence and voice. Her voice was—is—calm and slow, no hurry to it. It expresses no agenda, but accepts and responds to what is. And it is a kind voice, a soothing voice, voice as balm. That is a lot to ascribe to a voice, but such characteristics come through when it is all you have to go on.

But then there was also all of Edith sitting across from me, toes touching mine from time to time, as happens in a hot tub. It was too dark to make out a shape, but even more vivid than her voice was Edith's presence, a presence that easily conveyed who she was: compassionate, merciful, gracious. As we talked, relaxed and peaceful in the warm water and inky night, Edith asking pointed questions that called out who I was, she made me feel she was happy to know me. I felt welcomed, seen for who I was, seen even in total darkness. I was *apprehended*.

She told me she was a therapist with a Jungian orientation, and I tucked the information away for future use. Once a reference librarian, I still keep mental files because I like resources, I like connecting people with what they need, and I didn't know any Jungians in our immediate area. I was just visiting at the time; I had moved from western Massachusetts to New York to return to school, and I was back for a weekend of renewal, as I often was during those years. I did plan to return someday to do ministry, and for that reason I registered Edith's name as a possible referral source. And as a possible new friend.

There was no way of knowing at that time that I would crawl out of New York years later completely spent, exhausted beyond anything I had ever experienced or imagined possible, and in need of tender care. I remembered Edith, called her, and felt incredible relief and gratitude when she said she could see me. I knew she was sought by people throughout the country for teaching, workshops, and programs as well as by local people wanting her as a therapist. I began seeing her on a fairly regular schedule, punctuated by her trips around the country. Edith's office is in her home on Horse Mountain. I loved driving there, past a stunning birch tree at the edge of a cemetery, and then tunneling through the trees that surround her house and emerging into her space, where I was so warmly welcomed. Through several months Edith "held" me, her presence bringing me back to life, sustaining me, encouraging me, empowering me.

It was Edith *herself* who healed—and that is what she is, a healer. Healers take many shapes and use varied methods; their training can come with a Ph.D. or from a local school of massage. Or they may have none at all. In Edith's case, her credentials are sterling: teacher of philosophy at the University of Chicago, years of training in psychology, and now teacher, writer, advisor, therapist. Those experiences shaped her and gave her a form within which to work, a discipline. But once that is established, once one finds a hospitable theory or framework and learns it and pays one's dues, then all of the training falls into the background and the healer's authentic self emerges in the foreground, like chiaroscuro painting. The authentic self heals, and with just that self, Edith embraced me so that I could heal.

It was important to me that Edith could speak the language of theology and that she was trained in a discipline of which I had some understanding, psychology, and especially that she knew about midlife and what our psyches are calling upon us to do at this precarious and bedeviling time. We talked about all that, and much, much more, but her words have already faded from memory. What remains for me, what stands out in crisp clarity, is what Edith gave me through her presence, the very presence that drew me to her in the hot tub the first time I met her.

First and foremost was her attention, the kind of attention that focuses the moment and opens it up to all the richness that lies waiting in *any* moment if we can just attend. Developing such attention takes discipline and is at the same time a gift one is given. One can learn it, as in Zen meditation, with years of practice, but it is also something for which one must have a talent or at the very least a yearning. Edith has both. When she turned it upon me, I felt plunged into a place of succor so deep and so renewing that healing began to come upon me instantly.

In Edith's presence I felt seen. I knew she "got" me, saw me and took me in and mirrored me to myself. The self she saw was unique, with certain characteristics that only I carried. In Edith's eyes I had gifts to give the world, and the world would be the lesser for it if I didn't put them into action. We all need to be seen for who we are. We all need to be recognized. We all need to be urged to offer our gifts. We have been created as unique individuals, but so often lose touch with our centers, the part that makes us, us. To be seen and reminded of who we truly are is healing because it binds us back to that long-forgotten person, the original self. Rare are the persons who see this way and convey it. Edith does.

Edith's empathy, so full of tender mercy, is a third aspect of her presence. We know empathy when we feel it, but it's difficult to say what it is with any degree of exactitude. It's like having "attitude"—people have it or they don't, but we know the genuine thing when we see it. Edith has empathy, but I can't tell you more than that. I see it in her eyes, on her face, in the way her body responds to me even while sitting still. I feel it in her hug. She conveys the sense that I am okay, I am in fact fine, I have *standing* in some cosmic order. She never said any of that with words: it was all felt, transmitted by some means of communication that is Edith's, that is any healer's. I was its recipient, and weekly, it took hold in me, in my very cells, and remade my organism and healed what I didn't even know needed healing. Attention, the ability to see, and empathy: agents of healing, mediated through presence, Edith's presence. People have long found healing in pools of water—a hot tub, in the middle of an average American backyard, will do.

come into this room!

James 5:14–15 (one of the letters in the Christian Scriptures) advises us that if someone is ill, the elders of the church should be called in to pray over that person and anoint him or her. James doesn't instruct us to say prayers in church; he says the elders must be summoned to the bedside to pray and anoint the one who is ill. In other words, the elders must be *present*. There are many kinds of prayer, and any prayer is important to someone who needs healing. James is on to something important, though, that bears reiterating: human presence and human touch can have significant impact on healing when added to prayer. A person in the flesh, touching and praying, can have a powerful effect on anyone who stands in need of healing.

I absorbed the value of this bit of wisdom through experience as a hospital chaplain, for in that work, I discovered that presence and touch and prayer intentionally brought to bear on a situation in need of healing can bring healing where it seems impossible. I learned this most vividly when I was in training one summer at Columbia-Presbyterian Medical Center, New York City. We were a group of trainees, mostly seminary students, who provided pastoral coverage throughout the hospital. On call by beeper, a chaplain was summoned along with the medical team whenever someone was thought to be dying. My very first call as chaplain on duty was to the emergency room. I raced down to the ER, which was always packed full and usually chaotic, where a neurosurgical resident told me that an eight-year-old boy had been brought in by his mother in a taxicab, shot in the head by her former boyfriend. The boy had no chance of surviving, but the team was working on him, while his mother and aunt sat nearby in a closet of a room used for families in just such traumatic circumstances. I, the chaplain, had been called to comfort the family and to be with them when the awful news was delivered.

Opening the door to meet them, fear pounding in my heart, I was amazed to see two tiny girls—not women, girls—teenagers of indeterminate age, clinging to each other, as vulnerable as I had ever seen anyone look. They were in shock, obviously, and the mother's arms and clothes were covered with her son's blood. They were both clutching small gold crosses in their hands, crosses that must have been around their necks. I introduced myself, sat down, took the mother's hand, and had no idea what to do next. *Any* words I could think of seemed not only insufficient, but profane. What could I possibly say to comfort a child whose own child was lying in the next partition, dying of a gunshot wound to the head?

While I struggled to find some appropriate way to respond to them, the door was flung open by a large woman of color, about six-two, wearing shorts and a tank top. She filled the tiny room with her huge presence. She grabbed up the two sisters by crooking her massive arms around their necks and pulling them to her, calling them her babies. (She was, I discovered later, their neighbor.) And then in a commanding voice full of authority, she ordered Jesus to come into the room "right this minute, come in here, Jesus, my babies need you, and they need you *now,* I don't mean later, I don't mean in ten minutes, I mean *now!* Get down here! Come into this room and comfort these babies! Jesus, Jesus, get in here now.

There's nothing anyone can do but *you*." As I looked on with admiration and wonder, I felt the energy in the room change; a palpable sense of peace came over all of us. The mother stopped crying and moaning, and her breath slowed, became deeper, more even.

Their neighbor continued to hold the two girls in her mammoth, viselike elbows, rocking them both back and forth. I put my arms around them all and joined in the rocking. We swayed there together in one hot, sticky, bloody mass for ten or twenty minutes, I suppose. I had no sense of time or of place: all I felt was the love of this woman, and the love of God that she had so forcefully, and so effectively, called into the room. Once the peace had descended and the girls were noticeably calmed, the neighbor woman left, walking out as abruptly as she had come in, but the palpable sense of love and comfort remained long after the few minutes of her presence.

Healing? Absolutely—the most immediate, most effective, and most powerful I've seen. I am certain today, looking back, that what fueled her, what "made it happen" was that the neighbor was fully present, totally open, full of love and faith, and conveying all that through her body, which she used to hold and support the girls. She was *there,* as vividly present as a person can be, she summoned God there, and her presence, touch, and prayer invoked the healing needed at that moment. Everything was not all right. There was not a good ending; the boy died the next day. But God had been called upon and had been with the suffering mother and aunt, and they had felt God's presence, were able to function and get through that horrifying situation.

Had they been left alone, God forbid, or even with me, there with every good intention but not able to be present myself, overwhelmed as I was, the day would have been one of unmitigated horror instead of one where they were able to feel God-with-them. Healing can come in extraordinary moments we never forget, even when the conditions don't change. I cannot help believing that these two girls, women now, look back upon their neighbor's ministrations as what bound up that devastating crisis as much as it could be bound, as what made it bearable at that moment, even if it was unbearable during the years of grief that surely followed. Presence, touch, prayer—advised in the first century of Christianity, still workable some two thousand years later. A healing formula available through services of healing, through lay caregivers in a church, and through neighbors, ordinary people who have God's Spirit at heart and are ready to share it in extraordinary moments.

· 8 ·

church sanctuary

Tina St. Armand works in the office of a large church in lower
Fairfield County, Connecticut. She has worked there for ten
years, so she knows the congregation well, its families, history, traditions, politics. Over the years she has developed
into something of an institution, and anytime something
needs to be found out, tracked down, or remembered, Tina
is called upon, in part because of the breadth of her knowledge, and in part because she has an incredible memory,
somewhat like that of a computer: whatever she puts in there
for permanent storage stays and is quickly accessible to her.
Phone numbers, parkway exits, directions to any spot in New
England, dates of deaths and birthdays and baptisms, and
facts about people's lives (e.g., oldest daughter just moved to
Kalamazoo) are locked in her brain along with more spiritual
and psychological matters, such as who seems down, who is
facing serious surgery, who seems in need of a pastoral call.

Sitting at her desk greeting people, answering the telephone, working her computer, always doing at least three
things at once, and continually interrupted by the church
staff, she nonetheless manages to exude a peaceful, calm feeling that is catching. Tina, who looks much younger than
whatever her age, has an expressive, almost cherubic face,

rarely hiding what she feels (although she can do it when necessary), with dark eyes and a beatific smile. She is warm, inviting, friendly, and genuine, someone who is obviously at home in the place where she is and makes others feel the same way. All this makes her particularly well suited to the work she does as a general factotum of the church. But she has something more: she has the ability to heal by telephone.

Many of us conduct our lives through telephone (and other technology), and everyone has experienced what a difference the person on the other end of a telephone call can make simply through voice and presence. Getting a feeling for someone who is not there giving bodily cues depends on what she conveys with her voice and how genuine she sounds. I usually refuse the call when a telephone solicitor calls, yet I will sometimes pause and listen if a warm, friendly voice captures my attention. This happens rarely, but enough to know that voice makes a difference.

Tina takes calls all day long from members of the church as well as a range of other calls, people not affiliated with the church seeking help, and normal daily business. The calls from church members cover a vast array of possibilities: arrangements for a supper, inquiries about church school, calls to check whether someone is still in the hospital, calls from someone who is ill, lonely, or whose family member has just died. Tina needs to be able to react to what she has heard and what she is asked quickly, adeptly, call after call.

Her special talent is that in the midst of this busy office, with phones ringing, people talking, others wandering in and out looking for supplies, faxes, names, phone numbers, and typing assignments, she is able, most of the time (for she is not, after all, a saint), to stay calm and centered, making each caller feel that she or he is the only person who has called that day and that Tina has all the time in the world. She elicits their concerns with her obviously caring voice; she tends to the wounds; she soothes with her tender, genuine empathy. Listening with attentiveness, Tina makes a person feel heard, for indeed she *does* hear. She picks up on every nuance, every unspoken word, every shed or unshed tear. Her ability seems to be part attentiveness and focus, part intuition, part bringing to bear all that she knows about the context of situations, and certainly a large part, her capacity for empathy and sympathy. *Whatever* constitutes the mix, what is important is that people calling the church feel tended to, and I have heard, over and over again, that Tina makes people feel better after a brief telephone conversation.

She is able to touch people's neediness and loneliness. This particular church is in one of the most affluent areas in the country, but that does not mean its members are exempt from the human struggle. People there are not likely to admit to problems, but somehow, Tina manages to provide a snug, safe space there on the phone where they can give voice to what hurts. Tina provides *sanctuary*. There is, in that church, a large, modern sanctuary, with soaring ceiling and brick walls, a dramatic setting for worship. But creating a *feeling* of sanctuary requires human intervention, warmth, rich tone, a certain quality of absorbency, and that is what Tina offers in the office, as opposed to what can be apprehended in the sanctuary itself. Healing comes through God's presence, which can be found anywhere, anytime. As a member of the clergy, I fervently hope and pray that healing happens in sanctuaries, attended by ministers, but I know that we often fail at this task or simply let it go unaddressed.

Tina proves that healing can and does come wherever it will, in the office as well as the sanctuary, through the secretary as well as the minister. It is, after all, God who designates the capacity to heal, and in this church, God seems to have reached down the hallway from the sanctuary and tapped Tina, bestowing healing powers in an ordinary person, an ordinary place. The juxtaposition makes me see, once again, that healing happens where it will; it will not be confined to our ideas of it. It knows no borders, no "appropriate" settings. It awaits any who are open to it, in the moments that happen in ordinary days.

· 9 ·

imagine!

Easthampton, Massachusetts, is a town that was once prosperous. A manufacturing center for covered buttons, it also produced textiles and brushes in huge mills built of solid red brick. These fine buildings now stand empty, although in one of them craftspeople and artisans have pieced together studios, and another is in the process of being renovated for offices and apartments. Still, Easthampton has not enjoyed the same degree of successful revitalization as its neighbor Northampton has by renovating and restructuring its economic base. Northampton is hip, known for its creative and diverse populace, its arts, its restaurants and shops. Easthampton is stolid. So it is somewhat surprising that in the middle of downtown Easthampton there sits a tiny restaurant serving some of the best food to be found anywhere, food prepared and served by Jill Garfunkel, proprietor. Jill makes every morsel she serves, except for the bagels—homemade rye bread toast with scrambled eggs, chocolate cake, rugelach, chowders, roast chicken sandwiches, spicy shrimp, sautéed spring greens, pork loin with cherries, and more. Ingredients are for the most part local, including the eggs, and the menu reflects what is in season. The best bargain is brunch: a plate of fruit that might include fresh local strawberries or raspberries, a dish such as asparagus quiche (the nearby town of Hadley is known as the asparagus capital of the world), blueberry pancakes, or roast beef hash, fried potatoes, and bacon, $6.95.

Called Imagine, after John Lennon's song, Jill's restaurant contains six tables, plus a short counter that seats four. A simple and practical space, it is decorated with changing exhibits by local artists, a few odd pieces of cookware, and an assortment of plants, supplemented by bouquets from someone's garden, or potted hyacinths in March, when it is likely still winter in western Massachusetts and we are desperate for color and fragrance. A red-and-blue neon sign in the only window announces when Imagine is OPEN. Service is sometimes slow, depending on how many tables are filled, and whether or not someone is waiting tables. Sometimes Jill has to dash out of the kitchen (wiping her dough-spotted hands on the dishtowel wrapped around her waist) to take orders and pour coffee as well as prepare the food. Her partner, Joe LeGras, is sometimes in the kitchen, too, but he has other duties such as shopping and copying the menus that take him outside. Joe is tall and lean, wears a bandanna twisted around his head, and tends toward the irascible; his dark mutterings add a certain weight to the place that may in fact anchor it. There are also Luke, a gentle young man who brings a sense of calm, working as he does in sync with his own rhythm; Peter, gregarious, full of good humor, full of life; and others. It is the breakfast crew I know best.

Regulars are used to the slower pace, and if you were in a hurry, you would know there could be a risk in coming to Jill's that day. You do *not* want to hurry when you choose to eat there—the whole point is for your soul to be nourished, and the soul's pace is not a fast one. For better even than the scrumptious food served is the feeling of warm welcome Jill offers. Her cafe offers community and communion to the mismatched group who gather there to be fed, body and soul. Occasionally, I have been there when new customers come in (more this year since there have been two glowing restaurant reviews in regional papers)—easy to spot because they're usually "dressed" and appear by their demeanor to be from Boston or New York—and once or twice I've seen people stalk out because they weren't getting served fast enough. Their loss. To partake of Jill's food, a body needs to be patient and open and not of an irritable sort. The folks who end up there in a hurry are there simply to eat. The rest of us are there for more, and more or less know it, and we are willing to wait: we are there for soul food.

One Thursday morning my partner, Nancy, and I stopped by for a midmorning breakfast, wanting both food to eat and a peaceful place to do some planning for a liturgy we were to conduct that Sunday. As we entered, we were followed in by six to eight people, most of whom had some kind of developmental disability. Most likely they were from the sheltered workshop nearby. The group was noisy, a drink was spilled, and the din was punctuated by one woman who kept asking loudly for "Lunch!" every three or four minutes, even though her companion explained they were there for breakfast, not lunch. Jill looked a bit worried about the effect the ruckus might have on others, but she needn't have been. We all felt taken in, including, I'm certain, the group from the workshop, who must face all-too-common exclusion and shutting out in other places in their lives—but not at Jill's, for there an inclusive sense of community is created. There sanctuary is offered. *All* are welcomed at the table; *all* are fed the life-giving food.

Somewhere in her fifties, Jill has close-cropped hair and moves with smooth grace across the floor when she emerges from the kitchen to greet her customers. She was once a dancer, and some of the dancer's aura remains around her. She is "in her body." It is her face, though, that catches you up. Compassion shows all over her face; it shines from her eyes, eyes with a slightly sad cast to them, or the shadow of pain. Jill bears something, the weight of her life experience perhaps, or the gravity that can come with knowledge of human suffering. My suspicion is that she has done a lot of things in her day, been through quite a bit. She may wrestle with her own demons. I say that because she could not have developed the remarkable degree of compassion she has otherwise, and her compassion marks her as a healer, compassion so deep that it feels as though it has no limits, can stretch as far as it must to meet you where you are.

Her compassion is coupled with a remarkable intentionality, and the intention is clear: to welcome you as her guest. Radical hospitality, I would call it. Jill brings everything she has to bear on the moment in which you are in her care. Making a living as a chef seems irrelevant; in the moment of welcome, she seems more like a master Buddhist monk, piercing through everything to ask how things are. The restaurant is often busy, many things going on at once, but when Jill comes out from the kitchen and focuses on you, you feel her intentionality. She remembers what is going on in your life, and she asks about recent triumphs or losses. When she asks you how you are, she means it. When she asks if everything is all right, she means it. She is utterly genuine, and something about her presence pulls you out of wherever else you have been, or are going to, into the present moment. By being so utterly devoted to your well-being as her guest, so utterly present, Jill somehow stops the clock and enters with you into a timeless moment where all *is* indeed well. Her ability to connect is uncanny—she does it better than many therapists or ministers I know—and in that moment of connection, healing happens. You go from being a patron tucking in to the world's best pancakes to a member of a congregation about to receive communion from a celebrant who offers her entire self in the way Jesus wanted us all to do, by stepping into the timeless realm that he called the reign of God and reaching out to another human being in love. To be so met, even for an instant, is healing. That is one way (among others) Jesus healed, and it is a way that can heal today if we can find our way to people with such gifts.

Our souls long for such nourishing encounters, such feeding, but we find them rarely, looking for them where we think we *should* find them, like church, and all too often finding them missing, instead of being open to encounters in more ordinary places, like funky restaurants. Christians are taught that the sacrament of communion is conveyed through grace. But grace is not limited to working only through the ordained, at altars. Grace is not constrained. It works in its own ways, and clearly, grace is at work through Jill, who serves a bread of life of her own making. She is not saintlike or ethereal, far from it. She has bad days and bad weeks. She gets distracted; she worries about the business; she is an "ordinary" human with weaknesses along with her strengths. But she *does* have the extraordinary ability to enter into the moment, giving of her life energy to whatever she is doing, to such a degree that it can be tasted in her corn chowder, her carrot cake, her lamb chops, felt in the quality of her attention, seen in the gentle and generous treatment of all who come through her door. She embodies care and concern, mixes them into food, and serves them up for anyone choosing to partake. Bread of life, served on the corner of Union Street and Chapman Avenue, Easthampton, Massachusetts.

· 10 ·

finding a muse

In 1995 a wonderful biography of Ralph Waldo Emerson was published by the University of California Press, written by Robert D. Richardson Jr., entitled *Emerson: The Mind on Fire*. Among those who read, people sometimes cite titles of books that changed their lives. This book did something like that for me: it gave me a muse. And in finding my muse, which I had not known I lacked (or had been seeking), I regained a disenfranchised piece of myself, delivered back to me by RWE.

Emerson comes alive in this fine work. Richardson evoked his time, place, friends, intellectual companions, his family life with its many sadnesses, his struggle with and subsequent decision to leave the ministry he had practically been born to, his formulation of transcendentalism, his lecturing, and more so vividly that I felt I knew him well. But I wanted to know him intimately.

I read Emerson's essays and other work, found biographies and other resources written about him in various libraries, went to visit his home in Concord as well as his nearby grave. I have never had a particularly good imagination for history, rarely get much out of visits to historical sites, but there in Emerson's house I was thrilled to see his walking stick, his hat, his long black wool cloak. Besotted by Emerson I was. I loved the woodcut portrait of him that graced the cover of Richardson's book, and the artist, Barry Moser, happens to live in our area. My partner, Nancy, bought me that woodcut as a gift, among the best I've ever received!

In his preface, Richardson says that Emerson "never wrote for groups or classes or institutions; his intended audience was always the single hearer or reader." I know this to be true because I am a single reader who responded to Emerson with passion. His ideas, his message, went straight to my heart. I had read him much earlier in life, in high school and college, but I took him in on an entirely different level now, years later. As a preacher, I know that people respond to sermons because of what they bring to the sermons: something is going on within them, they need to hear a particular "word," and they receive what they need if the time is right. I needed, still need, to hear the word that Emerson so eloquently delivered because he speaks to my very soul. My intellect appreciates him, certainly, but it is my soul that he nourishes, my soul that needs the very word he has to give, my soul that feels as if it is being coated with a balm made from precious oils when I sit down with Emerson.

What I love and need and respond to in RWE is not important, really. What *is* important is the fact that such a thing can happen, this intense, soulful, fertilizing communion with a man long dead, but so alive for me. I do feel his spirit is available to me to inspire me and to guide me. When I gaze at his picture, which hangs on the wall above where I write, I see such kind and compassionate and deep eyes, such a modest, genuine, half smile. He had something extraordinary: a spirit unbounded by his time, an intellect steeped in God as well as in all things of the mind, a heart deeply schooled by both sadness and simple joys. All of that, and more, is somehow available to me still and inspires me to think deeply, to use my own experience, and to speak my own truth, as he did.

A muse is defined as the goddess or power conceived to inspire a poet (or other creator). My muse, Emerson, gives me power, making it accessible to me when it is not there for me to call up on my own, or so it seems. In Emerson I found a mentor capable of loosing the ties that keep me fettered, setting me free to create, to write, to be true to all that is in me. He is a kind of mirror through which whatever I see in him can also come into being in me. He holds a key for me, a key to unlock what is there, waiting. And in finding my muse (and such an unlikely one at that!) I can reclaim what belongs to me, what *is* me, and put it out into the world, when I might not be able to under my own steam alone.

Finding a way to reach into your interior and pull out what is there, especially if it has been there waiting to be brought forth, is healing. As Jesus said in the Gnostic Gospel of Thomas, "If you bring forth what is within you, what you bring forth will save you. But if you do not bring forth what is within you, what you do not bring forth will destroy you." A muse helps bring forth what is within you. A muse calls something into being. A muse makes manifest. A muse can come to you from anywhere, at any time. It doesn't seem to be in your control, but if and when it does appear, it wants you to respond to it and welcome it into your life. Finding a muse, finding any way to access the hidden stores of treasure that you have within, is a step in integrating your various parts into one whole being. Anytime you can bring back into your center a piece of yourself that has been off somewhere, lost, you are healed. Call it a muse, call it the Spirit of God, call it grace, but call it. Call forth what is within you. It can save you.

· 11 ·

a train ride

I enjoy the train and like taking it when I have the time, so on one occasion in the late eighties I purchased a ticket on Amtrak to go to Washington, D.C., for a speaking engagement in Virginia. I was looking forward to this particular trip with anticipation because I hadn't had time to myself for a while and I relished the idea of eight hours alone. With me I had two or three books, a few magazines, and my talk to edit. I also had a picnic lunch. The train didn't look crowded, so it seemed I would have the double seat to myself. I arranged myself for what I hoped would be a quiet and productive ride.

Having boarded in Springfield, Massachusetts, I had barely settled in when we stopped somewhere in Connecticut. I watched as the conductor led a disabled young man through the sliding doors that divide the cars. I had chosen a seat in the first row so I'd have room to stretch my legs. The conductor approached the empty seat next to me, all the while talking loudly to the young man as if he was deaf or mentally impaired or both. He sat him down next to me, shouting that he would tell the young man when we got to Philadelphia, where he would get off. I admit I looked on with growing dismay. Now I'd have someone next to me, someone who probably would need help, certainly not someone I could easily ignore, because his body jerked spasmodically. I saw my relaxing, cozy solitude disappearing before my very eyes, and I resented it.

Within a few minutes my new companion asked me a question, or so it seemed. I could *barely* make out what he was saying since his speech was drastically impaired; he spoke only with great effort and so slowly that one sentence took minutes to complete. With this new wrinkle I sank completely. To listen would take all my attention, all my energy, and certainly all my patience. But I knew I had to do it. I am good at doing what I perceive to be my duty, and it seemed my duty to listen, so listen I did. All the way to Philadelphia. By the time his stop rolled around, I looked up in surprise. So soon? I was enchanted, drawn into his story and bathed in his love. When he departed, I felt only gratitude at having been given such a great gift, his acquaintance.

Tony told me he lived with adoptive parents. He was eighteen and had come to the United States when he was ten, having been picked off the streets of Calcutta by Mother Teresa when he was an infant. Having been born with severe disabilities due to brain damage at birth, he had been abandoned, left on the street to die. But somehow he was found by Mother Teresa and reared in her orphanage. Mother Teresa educated him, having discovered that although he had physical disabilities, he had a fine mind. She had done the work, but Tony gave all the credit to God. His adoption by loving American parents was a miracle, he felt, and now that he was no longer a boy, he wanted to devote his life to God in thanks for all he had received. He wanted to be a priest, but had been turned down because it would be too hard for him to say the Mass. He then decided to become a brother in a monastery, where he could live a life of relative silence and his speaking disability would not present a problem—or so he thought. He had already been turned down twice by two brotherhoods who felt they could not admit him. I was incensed, shocked that religious orders could be so unseeing, unloving. Tony, however, explained that although he had been disappointed, he had total faith in God, and he knew that if God wanted him to be a brother, he would be one. The trip to Philadelphia was to yet another order. He was being interviewed for possible acceptance and would spend that day and night at the order. He asked me to pray for him, and I did, hard and fervently, over that day and the next.

Tony's faith was the most palpable I have encountered in anyone, and it coursed through his very being. I felt it. I took it in through my body and heart and soul. It was real. There was nothing righteous, or self-righteous, about Tony, nothing pious, no smacking of a "good" Christian. He was a human being who had every reason to feel sorry for himself or be embittered, and yet he was full of love and optimism, full of the Divine. For the first time I understood what it meant to be an old soul, for Tony was indeed an old soul, full of wisdom and mercy and kindness.

A few stops before he was to detrain he told me that he could make miracles happen by asking God to help people. He said his prayers were always answered, and he told me he wanted to ask God for whatever I wanted because I had given him a gift that day, the gift of attention. He said he rarely met anyone who took the time to listen to him, and therefore, he rarely felt seen for who he was. People were always in a hurry, he said, and it was impossible for him to hurry, so he was more or less confined to his family for relationships and discourse. They were wonderful, but he knew he had to make a life of his own, and he had just been praying to meet someone who would listen to him who didn't *have* to, but who just would. He had sat by me and his prayer was answered, he said. So, he asked, what did I need? What dreams did I have? I replied that I truly felt I had all I needed, that I couldn't think of a thing, but he pressed: "Anything, anything, ask for it and I'll pray, and you'll get it!" My trip was turning into a fairy godfather story: I believed him. The train slowed as it pulled into Philadelphia. I had this one chance, one wish. There *was* one thing I wanted, had wanted for as long as I could remember. I wanted to have a book published. I told Tony that was it, that was my heart's desire, and he assured me it would be mine. My book would be published. All I had to do was to write it.

The train stopped. I helped him up, hugged him, kissed him goodbye, and shed a few tears. I knew I would never see him again, and I would never know if he got to become a brother. I saw two monks waiting for him on the platform as he made his way slowly down the aisle, turned as he paused at the door, made a funny grimace at me—his smile—and stepped off and away.

And so it was that an awkward, orphaned stranger on Amtrak taught me two very important lessons about healing. The first is that healing always involves a mutuality of some kind. The energy of healing doesn't simply flow from one person into another—it moves back and forth between the two (or more). Even when one person is designated as the one needing healing, the other is receiving as well as giving: receiving renewed energy, an opened heart, love. The second thing I learned from Tony was about attention. There is something in the very act of attending to someone that focuses energy, and such focused energy can heal. To be healed, one must be attended to; focus, energy, love, any or all of these must be brought to bear by oneself or by a healer. A response must somehow be catalyzed and something or someone must act as the catalyst. I had given Tony my attention, and he responded. He gave me his, and I responded. There was something healing for both of us in our encounter, and the mutuality of attention was the agent.

· 12 ·

touch

Many types of bodywork are now practiced, each with its own theory or tradition behind it. By "bodywork" I mean any method of working directly on the body for therapeutic purposes. No matter what the theory behind a particular school of bodywork, it is a way for people to be touched, and we all need touch. Touch, in and of itself, can be healing. Bodywork is a way to be touched in a professional manner in a society that has become suspicious of touch, necessarily so, in many cases. But human beings need appropriate touch, even if we are not consciously aware of it, and will find ways to get it in positive, healthy ways or not-so-healthy ways.

In the past, not long ago, healing by touch was conveyed by physicians and was, I suspect, an important component of what was called bedside manner. An empathic doctor sitting by the bed, listening to the patient while holding a hand or touching an arm, held the power to heal. Now that most doctors don't have time to sit with someone in their office for ten minutes, let alone make house calls, such healing has become an anachronism in the medical community, and that may have something to do with why more and more people are turning to bodyworkers for what they need.

A person doesn't have to know or believe in the theory underlying any particular type of bodywork to benefit from it. Some types come from centuries-old tradition, others have been developed in recent years, and a few may have little or no theory behind them at all. While the theory may matter little to the person being worked on, it can be important to the practitioner, giving structure, technique, and a group of professional colleagues. What seems most important, however, is the practitioners themselves and their ability to spark a response within the body. I know three bodyworkers, each quite different from the others, each from different schools of practice, who have the ability to heal, and what they have in common is that each conveys something through touch that enables the body to right itself.

Renee Gorin is a bodyworker in New York City whom I met while I was interim seminary pastor at Union Theological Seminary. The seminary pastor serves as the minister to the school community of some four hundred people and has responsibility for the spiritual well-being of that community. Working with students of all ages going through life changes, seekers on spiritual journeys, brilliant young scholars preparing to teach theology and biblical studies, renowned faculty members, and creative and dedicated staff, I cannot imagine a congregation richer, deeper, or more varied than this one.

Seminary can be difficult, and I spent a good deal of my time counseling students. Everyone had his own measure of pain to bear, her own issues to work out. A steady stream of suffering flowed through the office. As time went on, I felt that suffering settle on my shoulders, a heavy mantle that seemed to work its way into my body. In the fall of my second year I was seized with a flulike illness and couldn't shake it; it was with me six, eight, ten weeks. My predecessor had been attacked by severe arthritis her second year into the job and had been unable to work for several months. So it didn't take me long to realize that my illness had something to do with the job, and that I needed help. I turned to my friend and colleague Margaret Kornfeld, a pastoral psychotherapist.

Margaret, in her wisdom, recommended that I see a colleague of hers, Renee Gorin, who did bodywork. I trust Margaret, so I called Renee for an appointment and went to see her, even though I wasn't sure of what I was getting into.

Renee's office is almost square, a plain room in the Shaker sense, simple and clean. It is not large, but it felt ample, proportionate to the task, and in it was Renee, a small, perfectly proportioned woman. Renee and her space together conveyed a sense of rightness, of perfect "fit." Down her erect back hung a braid of grayish brown hair that looked as if it served as a plumb line, so centered was she in her body, so perfectly balanced. Renee seemed to be lined up with the axis of the earth and in harmony with all around her. Being in Renee's presence gave me a sense that I was "at home" and that with her I would find a place of repose. I began seeing her regularly.

Renee's work is not associated with a particular tradition; she has created her own technique. Through a combination of movement, touch, breathing, and imaging exercises, she brought me into her field of energy and let me rest there. For example, from time to time I would go into a deep, trance-like state brought on simply by listening to Renee's breathing, which was deep and tidal, while she worked. Her breath set up a rhythm that carried me with it into profound relaxation, a rest so restorative that an hour of it felt like a month's vacation at the seaside. Before long I shed what had accumulated in my body. The illness evaporated, but I kept going because Renee had begun to lead me more deeply into a sense of my body.

The men and women I worked with at Union were engaged in life-and-death struggles, for they were being remade in the crucible that is seminary. The depth and breadth of the students' journeys and the intellectual energy required to study theology were always incredibly intense. Anyone privileged to share the journey with them, as I was, could not avoid the intensity and be helpful—I had to go with them to be able to offer any comfort, any sustenance, any release. To traffic in such circles of the soul, I had to be conscious and clear and strong, able to take care of myself as well as others. Renee helped me discover that my boundaries (where I ended and someone else began) were quite permeable—I literally took in whatever someone I was with put out. Not being conscious of what was happening, I had done nothing to defend myself or to clear it out of me later on. Suffering, illness, psychic turmoil, and pain washed over me daily, and daily I had unknowingly taken it all into my body. Renee helped me to be aware of another person's energy and the responses it was causing in my body. She taught me how to maintain a less permeable membrane around myself, how to protect myself and not take in what was not mine. If I had not found Renee, I feel sure I would have soon sunk under the weight of it all; certainly, I could not have long continued in such work, at Union or elsewhere.

By healing me, Renee taught me something I urgently needed to learn, most of it centered on becoming conscious of my body, its messages and needs. I learned that the body has a consciousness of its own, and I can depend on it to give me cues to what is going on, both inside me and out. I learned not to treat this essential part of my self as an old workhorse, but to honor it. Responding to its clear messages, I eventually changed my diet, cut down on caffeine, began an exercise program, found I needed sun and air and being outdoors every day. My body has always been sensitive, but I had never heeded it. Once I did, I was able to use it properly in my work as a minister without sacrificing my own health and well-being.

Being with someone who is fully in her body, as Renee is, who connects with people, the earth, and the various energies in which we all live and breathe and have our being, heals. Renee's body, like that of anyone, is an instrument. Unlike most of us, though, her instrument is finely tuned, cared for, and practiced upon. Being so attuned, Renee is able to work from her body with others, person to person, body to body, energy to energy. Using her body, she sparked renewed life into me like she was jump-starting an old battery. Sometimes healing happens this way; the life force is taken in directly from the body of another. Sometimes we may not even know it has happened: it may be a quick touch, a hug, or a chance meeting with someone who radiates life. However it may come, we do well to understand that such healing forces are always around us, in many and varied shapes and places and people, capable of renewing us if we are willing to say yes to them. Renee shows how to say yes.

Shiatsu massage is a school of bodywork originating in Japan, based on the same tradition as acupuncture, which holds that a life force called Qi runs through our bodies on pathways called meridians. Qi is the force that binds everything together, and everything is infused with Qi. When it flows freely, we have a sense of balance and health. If the flow is blocked or disrupted, by bad dietary practices, stress, or injuries, for example, imbalance and ill health occur. Shiatsu focuses on prevention, for if your energy flows smoothly, you have a better chance of maintaining health. Shiatsu means, literally, "finger pressure," and the practitioners use their fingers, elbows, even knees, to apply pressure on these points.

A person need know nothing about shiatsu massage to experience its healing effects as practiced by Stevie Converse, shiatsu masseuse and teacher. Stevie (born Stephanie) works out of a studio in an old mill building undergoing renovation, having recently moved her office from downtown Northampton because she needed more space for the classes she teaches. Stevie's space is inviting; with pale walls and north light coming through the enormous windows, it soothes as soon as you enter it. This is not left to chance. Physical space is important in shiatsu, the color tone and positioning helping to create balance. (Physical space has long been considered an important element of healing, from ancient Greece, where those wishing to be healed went to the temples of Asclepius and walked labyrinths and slept on special dream couches, to the sanatoriums of the late nineteenth and early twentieth centuries located in mountains with plenty of sun and fresh air.)

Stevie is a smart, witty, dynamic woman of multiple talents. She is possessed of a strong sense of curiosity, which may have something to do with her range of talents. She gets sparked by something, learns all about it, and incorporates it into her world. Not surprisingly, her worldview is large and embracing, and life itself seems to provide her with plenty of kicks. Certainly, she is usually able to laugh about life, its twists and turns, even at some really bad points in her own. The agenda of things she'd like to do, try, create, far outstrips her life span, I have no doubt. One thing can be counted on with Stevie. If you ask her, "What's new?" two or three things always are. Her curiosity, her vitality, the sense she gives off that she is really enjoying living her life, all contribute to her magnetism. Her own Qi must be quite strong and balanced, for she is a walking advertisement for her practice.

Stevie maintains her shiatsu practice, teaches courses to aspiring practitioners, and travels widely to give workshops and seminars in shiatsu. She is also a cabaret singer with a powerful "Broadway" voice who is part of a trio (Le Cabaret) that entertains in New England. She used to sing solo in clubs in New York City (which is where she trained for shiatsu with her teacher, W. Ohashi), and she still does occasional solo gigs as time allows. In a recent show, Stevie did smashing imitations of Arthur Godfrey, Judy Garland, and Peggy Lee, having studied their voices and mannerisms on tape at the Performing Arts Library at Lincoln Center. But when doing shiatsu, Stevie is completely herself, authentic and true.

A shiatsu client lies fully clothed on a mat on the floor while Stevie moves around the mat on her knees, holding, pushing, pulling, and attending the body's responses. She works skillfully, adeptly, confidently. Stevie inspires trust, and that is important to the body's responses. We tend to hold in or back when we don't trust someone, relax when we do, and the relaxation response engendered by any bodyworker, including Stevie, is an important part of healing, for a rigid, tightly held body is not likely to take in healing properties: the "yes" response is necessary.

Rhythm is the thread tying together Stevie's massage practice and life as a troubadour. Immersed in rhythm, in the world of music, she works in response to her own rhythm and helps her clients get in sync with theirs. Rhythm is another way of describing the pulse of life, the force that runs through us, and she works with that in shiatsu, feeling the meridian points, determining what is sluggish, what blocked, what racing. Is the body's energy moving harmoniously, or is it off the beat? Stevie is a serious practitioner who has a great store of knowledge about her subject, and she has a great deal of experience that she brings to bear with any client. Where and how she touches may be based on the tenets of shiatsu, but the essential component seems to be her own touch. Perking with life, tuned in to her own rhythm as well as her client's, sensitive to the energies in and around us, Stevie heals by listening to the beat of life and then orchestrating it like a conductor, swaying, tapping, embracing the body's music, which she hears so precisely. With the help of someone like her, we can learn to feel our own rhythms and let life flow freely in us; we can come to a greater portion of wholeness.

Rosen method is a school of bodywork developed and taught by Marion Rosen. Rosen, now in her eighties and living in Berkeley, California, was—is—a physical therapist who originally worked on people's injuries. Folks kept coming back to her even after their injuries had healed, simply because it felt so good to be worked on by her. Over many years—and she has practiced her craft for more than sixty years now—Rosen slowly worked out a technique designed to relax tightly held muscles where feelings are stored. By letting go of what we have been holding in our muscles, our bodies and our energy are freed for use in more creative, life-giving ways.

The technique used in Rosen method bodywork is touch; some kneading, similar to massage, is done, but simple touch of the tight musculature is the main method, carried out on a person lying on a massage table, undressed except for underwear. The practitioner will also ask questions about or affirm what she notices happening in the body she is working on, to deepen the client's awareness of what is happening, to meet the client wherever she or he is. It is not interpretive, as in many kinds of therapy, but simply attentive: "Ah, yes, something just changed. Do you know what it was?" Such attention helps the client to focus on the feelings in her body and come to know her body/self in a new way.

That's the theory. The practice itself, conducted by the hands of a master, is so revivifying as to make you feel like you are being raised from the dead. The master is Joyce Loughran, a youngish, tidily compact woman whose demure appearance belies the fact that she is possessed of an extraordinary power—the power to heal with touch. Extraordinary talent in an ordinary person: as with other healers and modes of healing encountered, it is the very ordinariness that surprises. No bolts from the blue here. Rather, slow, steady applications of gentleness, conveyed through touch, voice, and presence.

Joyce is also a painter, and she brings an artist's sensibility to a client in that she seems to be able to see something more. She sees what places need touch; she sees where feelings and memories are held; she sees what is bound and needs loosening. And she seems to see beyond the flesh in hand to the greater possibilities inherent in a body—the creative openings that await us all if we were not so tethered to the various pains of our past or present. Joyce can alchemize a numbed body into something alive, inspirited, golden. To bring life back to where it is missing is the mark of a healer; Joyce does this through touch, using Rosen method as the way in, but again, her individual approach matters.

In Joyce's case, it is the quality and depth of her gentle respectfulness that heals. Whether it is through her quiet, deliberate movements, her silky voice, her skilled hands, or just her presence, she conveys the message that your body—you—are deserving of compassionate attention and respect simply because you are alive. Having compassion and respect for all is the message of great religious leaders, but so few of us ever get to feel it deeply, in our bones, in our lifetimes. We may be well treated because of status, power, or products we create, because of what we *do* in the world, but that is part of the quid pro quos that the world runs on; it has little to do with who we inherently *are*. Joyce offers an entirely different kind of respect, and it is there for anyone coming to her. Name, status, product, class, abilities, whatever definitions are applied to us by the world as a way to distinguish ourselves from one another, none have bearing in Joyce's presence. She truly offers a pearl of great price because it is so rare. I am someone who has had a measure of worldly respect, grown up with privilege, been treated with dignity, but my dry bones soak up what Joyce gives because I have not experienced it elsewhere, certainly not at such a profound level. It is what my soul desires: consideration merely for being me, nothing else required. Joyce witnesses to all life, to me as a particular expression of life, and that witness nourishes every cell in my body. It heals.

Such respectful witness also brings forth truth. Attended to thus, my body tells me what I need without the interference of my brain chattering away, schooled as it is to talk me into someone else's idea of what is right or wrong for me. Conformity has no purchase here; social approbation means nothing and easily slides away in the face of my body's own truth. Truth heals by cutting to the essential and recalling us to who we are and who we were meant to be. Finding our true "home," fitting, finally, into that long-sought spot, ah, how deliciously liberating and health giving *that* is!

To come down in the place just right, as the Shaker song goes, to find the place where we belong, to feel our inner and outer worlds move together in one integrated whole, that is healing on the deepest level. Through her touch, guided by her method, Joyce Loughran effects such changes and more. While certainly an extraordinary healer, Joyce is one bodyworker among many. If we are willing to open our bodies to appropriate professional touch, healing awaits us.

· 13 ·

"kitty spice"

We have a program in the church I serve that is part of a nationwide network called Stephen Ministry. People of the church are trained, and rather extensively so, to give care, primarily through listening, to others in the church and community. Our program is quite successful, a large one, and we do quite a bit of our work outside the church, in the greater community. So it was not unusual when I got a call to talk with someone I didn't know who might benefit from such care.

That's how I met Lee Berentsen. Suffering from devastating neurological complications from a virus, probably late-stage Lyme disease, she had been in and out of intensive care units, hospitals, and rehabilitation centers over a period of four or more years, nearly dying more than once. In her forties, Lee could hardly walk, used a cane, had lost memory, slept hours and hours at a time, but never really felt rested. She had lost her own, very successful business, since she could no longer work, had lost her home and former "friends." Yet in the midst of this Joblike story she was still able to laugh despite her tears, was getting herself moved to a new place, and had all the markings of a real survivor. What I saw behind the illness and its symptoms was one incredibly strong, magnetic, powerful woman. Parts of her body might have been broken, but she, I sensed, was whole in some deep part of her being where it really counts. How did she do it?

She told me during that visit that she played the piano and had trained as a younger person to become a concert pianist.

One of her many concerns involved her piano, which had been damaged when the ceiling fell through in the rented house where she was living. She told me she played when the labyrinth was set up to be walked in our church, which was how she knew our church. But I got no real sense at that time about the intense role music played in her life. On another visit, after she had moved to a new place, she told me about a music group she worked with called Music for People, a group important to her because it was a time to get together with other musicians and play. Again, it was a brief part of the conversation, brought up, I think, because she was hoping to be able to attend a weekend with them. I do remember her saying that music was the only thing that was keeping her alive.

Not long ago, the labyrinth was going to be set up at church for the fall equinox, fortuitously on a day when I would be there (I work at the church part-time). The labyrinth I refer to is a canvas copy of one that is designed into the floor of Chartres Cathedral, copied and made popular in this country by the Reverend Lauren Artress of Grace Cathedral, San Francisco. Various groups and churches now have their own copies, and it is laid out so that people can walk it as a spiritual exercise, as they did in medieval times in lieu of a pilgrimage. I went down late in the afternoon to the sanctuary and joined the group who were walking. The sun was setting, candles were set up on the edges, and to one side the piano and a cello were being played. I was immediately struck by the music, which was hauntingly beautiful. As I walked, spiraling in toward the center, each time I passed by the piano I looked at the woman playing: could this be Lee? She looked totally different from the last time I had seen her. I was confused because she looked so good, so peaceful, so intent! Finally, she winked at me, and I knew it was Lee. She played that day for six hours, just a few weeks after having had surgery on her wrist for carpal tunnel syndrome. She and the cellist played in a way I had never heard music played. The expression, the beauty, the mystery, the tone, all worked together to touch each one of us there in a profound way, I have no doubt.

Because I had not seen Lee in some time, I made an appointment to visit her a week or two after the labyrinth experience. I went to her home and found her ensconced in a comfortable chair next to the piano (recently renovated), her cat on the footstool on which she rested her legs. I asked her immediately about the labyrinth music. She told me that it had been six hours of improvisation, and that she and the cellist had not played together before. I found that hard to believe, but she went on to tell me about the Music for People group that she had mentioned to me some time ago. Founded by the cellist David Darling, this nonprofit foundation sponsors workshops in improvisation for both talented musicians and nonmusicians. Lee meets with them to play together, and she also works with the group as a teacher in training. Her long-range goal is to make music with people who are ill or dying, passing along what was given to her.

Nearby her, Lee had a compact disc of improvisational chamber music recorded at a Music for People workshop in 1997. As the insert to the CD says, what these people share is "a belief that the beauty of music lies in its power to connect humans to each other—by listening, by imitating, and by speaking their truth in sound. . . . Participants receive training in improvising for self-expression, developing their solo power to make authentic sounds, while honing their sensitivities for listening and blending." The recording was made from people given twenty minutes in a studio to play, solo or with others, with no rehearsals and no retakes.

Lee turned on the CD player. She played the work of a woman who is not a singer, someone who sat down at the piano to play and sing. The music was incredible. It was the most authentic human sound I have ever heard. It felt as though it came straight from that woman's soul into mine. That cut was followed by one of an Irishman singing gospel, and then by one of Lee herself playing piano and singing (which she doesn't "do" either) a piece called "Kitty Spice," inspired by a cat who visited her while she was bedridden. Those were but three of seventeen pieces of improvised music, the likes of which I have never heard. The sound was so genuine and true and beautiful in each of the selections that I could respond only with tears, followed by deep silence. I am sensitive to any energy that promotes healing, and I felt the familiar sensation move through me. This music has the power to heal. It may be just because it *is* so authentic and deep, and has the power to contact one's center. And one's true center *is* whole and complete. We so rarely have contact with it that we don't know the ecstasy of completeness that resides there.

I knew in that moment that this music must sustain Lee. Through this music, she is able to go into a place that is entirely whole, full of power, and transformative by its very nature. In this place, Lee is whole and healed: that was clear. It is not a place where she can stay all the time. No one could; it's too intense. It can be visited only for moments, but the moments are healing ones. This music does indeed connect humans to each other. I felt threads spun between the musicians and myself, and between Lee and me, pulling us together in the vast human enterprise. To be able to connect in such a way with any other human being is stupendous: soul to soul, center to center, life to life. It is that very connection that heals. It is mutuality at its most intense, powered by sound coming, it seemed, straight from the Source of life itself. Contact at the deepest center of the soul and, thankfully, available to anyone.

· 14 ·

daily walks

Beauty heals. This sounds too simple to be true in this day, at the end of the twentieth century in the United States, but it is. Beauty heals. I know this because I have been healed so, body and soul and psyche feeding on the beauty around me in great gulps after years of starvation.

I left western Massachusetts in 1989 to attend Union Theological Seminary in New York City. I had planned to go to seminary in Boston so that I could work out some sort of commute and remain in the Pioneer Valley (where I lived then and now), but it was Union that called to me, Union that was my fate. Despite all my misgivings, and there were many, I departed for New York, leaving behind my two hundred-year-old home, its view of Mt. Tom from the back of the property, the perennial gardens. I moved to a small two-bedroom apartment in school housing on the corner of Broadway and West 122nd Street. There were windows on two full sides, including one facing north, so there was wonderful light, but also incredible noise, including that from the M4 and 104 bus stop directly below.

Within a month of the move I ended up at the Columbia University Health Service having my inner ears examined because I thought I must have an ear infection, my equilibrium was so disturbed. I tripped for no reason walking down the street, sometimes missed a last stair step, and often felt "off balance." The doctor found nothing, and sometime later I realized what was not a medical condition was, in fact, a powerful symbol. I *had* lost my equilibrium, psychically, and I was feeling the effects, physically. I eventually stopped tripping, but I never did feel I regained my balance. New York, its energy, its noise, its gray stone and concrete so chilling in winter and so hot in summer, threw me off center. There were also its marvels, its creativity, its diversity, its aliveness: all of that is true, too, and I don't regret going, but the cost was high and left my soul bankrupt.

Before New York I was unaware just how much my environment mattered to me. Because I had never lived in harsh places, cleanliness and order and beauty were things I took for granted. Once they were missing I was surprised to feel such agony in their absence. I remember getting a paper back from a professor I respected, a paper on dreams. She wrote in the margin "Sounds as if you're starved for color!" I read that, let it sink into my bones, and it hit home—yes, yes, I was starved and didn't know it! New York was gray, and it was turning my soul gray. I tried to remedy this symptom of soul sickness by going to museums. I didn't care who the artist was, what the exhibit; I just wanted color, the more vivid, the better. The roof garden of the Met offered views of the greens of Central Park, and the herb garden at the Cloisters was balm for the eye with its subtle shades of mauves and blues and silvers. Only a year or two before leaving the city I discovered the glorious community gardens, riotous with color, in lower Riverside Park, not far from the Seventy-second Street boat basin. Color *can* be found in New York, but getting to it takes effort and usually costs money.

Color was one thing I needed, as were quiet; the smells of fallen leaves and wood burning, of country grasses and hays and lavender hot from the sun; the sights and sounds of animals and birds, especially hummingbirds with their iridescent blues and greens glinting in the sun; butterflies, flowers, trees, leaves, frogs croaking at night in spring and crickets chirping in August; the soothing proportions of old churches and houses and barns built to human scale and preserved and cared for; the order of neat woodpiles and clotheslines and vegetable gardens, laid out in rows.

All that was returned to me when I left New York after six years, coming home to western Massachusetts, finally, one September. Here, in fall, I am dazzled by the flaming reds and yellows of the huge old maples that line our street and cover the surrounding hills. There are the bright orange berries on the bittersweet vine that grows next to our little library (and sold for four dollars for a stem or two on corners along Broadway!) to which I walk two or three times a week to collect the books I've requested on interlibrary loan and to chat with our marvelous librarian. Walking daily, I see plump pumpkins in fields, and the purples and yellows of goldenrod and asters, all the more beautiful in contrast to the browns and grays of the fields in which they stand. An apple orchard is laden with fruit, ripe and soon to be turned into cider and pies. Freshly relined with straight, white lines, our street is striking in its cleanliness, the absence of litter startling to one who walked down dirty sidewalks every day for years. In the garden, chrysanthemums send out their pungent smell; it mixes with the clovelike scent of the last few old roses and that of the occasional stalk of lavender, which is about all that's left in the garden by now. Feeding outside the kitchen window where I sit at my computer are bright yellow finches, crimson cardinals, azure jays, red, black, and white woodpeckers. The crickets started chirping in August, always a melancholy sound to me because it means summer is nearly over, and a few weeks ago I heard an owl hooting outside the bedroom window late in the night.

There are no mesas or high mountains or canyons here, no drama to this countryside, but a gentleness, a merciful harmony to the hills, the buildings, the vegetation. My feet touch ground rather than concrete, my hands can dig in rich, dark earth, and every day my senses are filled with satisfying smells, sounds, tastes, sights, touch. There is no grayness now, though it will come in February and March—and then my soul will sputter and complain—but the grayness will also depart in due season, as it does every year. My soul knows that and trusts in the cycles of which I am a part. There is less harshness here, though hardiness is required. There is no continuous noise, though Saturdays are filled with the din of chain saws, leaf blowers, mowers, gun shots from hunters in November, and soon enough, snowmobiles. It is not paradise, but close enough to it to heal.

It is healing because human beings need to be connected to the life force, and the beauty of nature is one place to feel that force. Observing what is around me, paying close attention to what gives growth, learning the habits of the birds and bugs, taking in the beauty to be found just outside the door, all these are ways in which I can experience myself as a part of the larger scheme of things. A small part, but nonetheless a part, and so connected to life itself, and whatever it is that constitutes the mysterious force that both creates and destroys life. I cannot explain it, nor shall I try. I only know it, and I know that when it flows freely, and I am in it, and it in me, I am alive. I am as I was created to be, I am whole: I am healed. Beauty carries life's energy in its very being, and anyone who experiences beauty can be healed by it if conscious of it and open to it in whatever moment it is revealed.

· 15 ·

hilltown woman

Joyce Freeland is a woman of remarkable generosity of spirit who lives in a rural area of Massachusetts called the Hilltowns, small towns scattered through the foothills of the Berkshires. After a career in Washington, D.C., where she was the director of finance for the National Foundation of the Arts and Humanities (now the two national endowments), Joyce moved to Plainfield, Massachusetts. There she set up a financial management services business, working with nonprofits and small businesses. She was attracted to Plainfield's agrarian nature because she grew up on a farm in Indiana. She fits in well in her town, straightforward, confident, modest, and genuine as she is, as well as handy and strong. She knows how to hay, drive and fix tractors, cut wood, pull cars out of ditches in the snow. Now in her sixties, she sometimes forgets that she might need to slow down, as she did not long ago when she was visiting her sister Janet and tore down a garage using a sledgehammer as her tool of choice. She was achy on her return but couldn't figure out why, because she didn't consider sledgehammering a building to pieces anything out of the norm for a sixty-six-year-old woman!

There is another Joyce, the one her friends and neighbors don't know as well because we rarely see her in this role, and that is the one who traveled widely to developing countries, where she designed financial systems and audited research grants on children's medical issues given by the National

Academy of Science in such places as Bangladesh, Egypt, Senegal, Kenya, the Philippines, Ecuador, and Uruguay, more than thirty-seven countries in all, usually working in conjunction with a university there. Coming and going all the time for years eventually took its toll because the work was exhausting, so she travels less now, concentrating her energy on more local projects, such as working with the Hudson River Foundation and Woods Hole Research Center.

Over the years, Joyce has done an incredible array of work, starting out as a typist for the FBI when she graduated from high school, later selling knives door to door, waiting tables, and selling real estate when she was working her way through college at night to become a CPA. Whether she is working in the corridors of power in Washington, D.C., selling a product, or setting up an accounting system for a local folk singer, work is central to who she is in terms of no job being too small (or too large). Perhaps because she has done so many kinds of work, however, she is not defined by it, and it does not determine anything about her life other than providing money. Unlike many people whose self-concept is shaped by the power and status inherent in their jobs, Joyce simply does what she has to do to get by, and work serves her, not vice versa. In her day, she has had plenty of money, and she has had little. And never has it made a difference in how she lives her life.

It *has* made a difference in her ability to share whatever she has. Joyce never hesitates to help someone in need. In my experience, people who have money are less likely to give it than those who know what it is to be without, and who are therefore capable of relating to someone in need. Joyce lives in both camps, having money and having little, and unlike most, whether she has some money or very little, she is generous with whatever she has.

Whether the help is in time, goods, services, or money, she reaches into her deep stores of generosity and gives whatever there is to give, no promises necessary in return other than asking the recipient to pass it along to the next person, so that the same resource stays in constant circulation, going to whoever needs it next. (I know this because Joyce paid for my partner's son Chris to get periodic massages when he had cancer. Chris wanted to repay her somehow, but she asked only that he provide for someone else someday when he is in a position to do so.) She shares just as readily when she has no money as when she has plenty, when she has no time as when she has extra, even when it means she may be dropping into bed exhausted at 1:00 A.M. and getting up at 4:00 A.M. to drive to Bradley Airport in Hartford to fly to yet another country. Cleaning out a barn, taking a grandnephew fishing, helping a neighbor with haying, buying dinner for an underemployed friend, going to three church services in one day to support the worship leaders, helping someone trying to start a business, making an extraordinary number of phone calls weekly in order to stay in touch with various people needing support—all this and much, much more makes up the fabric of Joyce's life. Always approachable for yet another request for help, yet another call, yet another trip into town to meet a friend who needs an attentive ear, Joyce, more than anyone I know, doles herself out lavishly without regard to tomorrow, in the spirit Jesus recommended to us.

What feels best about being the recipient of her largesse is not so much the thing received as the spirit with which it is given. No judgment about whether money will be used wisely, no parsimony, no effort at control accompanies any of her gifts. They are pure gift—given only because Joyce can, and wants to, and does. It is all that is behind her gifts that counts most. It is, in fact, healing because she is sharing her own being, her own life, life itself, given directly from her to you. The thing being given is merely a symbol of the true gift, the gift of life and love, poured out with a generosity that knows no bounds. The recipient receives something that works on the heart and soul, and is transformative.

In the presence of such generosity, it is difficult to remain tight: generosity causes tightness to open like a moonflower reacts to darkness. It puts love into action, calls out similar action in response, looses a different, positive energy into the world. All this heals because it adds to our *common* wholeness. It's an adding in to the world rather than a taking from. When so much of life seems to revolve around getting, a generous spirit such as Joyce's frees us to live differently, to live from a truer center. When we recognize what we have been given, we *want* to pass it along. Someone must start that chain reaction, though, and Joyce is one such someone. In her generosity, she gives healing. I am sure there are others, riding tractors, passing through airports, fishing with children. They *can* be found, and what they have to give is nothing short of the gift of a more abundant, whole-making life.

· 16 ·

riding at mount holyoke

The Pioneer Valley Therapeutic Riding Association is a group of "horse people" who have banded together to provide riding lessons to people with various disabilities who might benefit by it. Both Mount Holyoke College and the University of Massachusetts volunteer their horses and stables to the venture, and instructors work with a team of volunteers who help groom, saddle, and walk the horses. (I am a walker at the Mount Holyoke site. I often walk with Sarah, a twelve-year-old who is home-schooled and does this work as part of an animal husbandry unit. Her aunt works in the stables at Belmont, so she knows a thing or two about horses.)

The stables are relatively new, clean and orderly and very well maintained and run. It is a pleasure just to walk inside and see that the horses are so well tended. Many of them belong to students at the college, which is known for its equestrian team, but others belong to the school, and they are the ones the program uses. My favorite is Cina, a big (both tall and wide) chestnut mare who is gentle and kind but also lively enough to provide a good ride. In fact, the college uses Cina to teach vaulting: students learn to propel themselves onto her back while she is cantering in a circle. Her height and broad back make her perfect for Sam, the young man who rides her while I walk alongside, with a fellow volunteer, in case he should begin to fall. Sam is a student at the University of Massachusetts in his early twenties, originally from

Brooklyn, who suffered a brain tumor in his teens. It was successfully removed in a daring, extremely delicate operation, but he was left with problems of balance, impairment in walking for which he uses assistance, slurring of speech. His mind is fine, however, and he has a quick and New Yorky sense of humor (wry, ironic, earthy). He is a hefty man, and mounting Cina can take some doing. Once he is up, he has a tendency to sway alarmingly in the saddle due to his problems with balance and weight distribution, which means the walkers beside him must really pay attention. But astride Cina, Sam really shines: he is confident, knows how to handle her, and is able to get the exercise that would be hard to come by otherwise.

Other riders include Jack, a man in his thirties who has cerebral palsy and must be lifted onto his horse, his severely contracted leg muscles so tight that his legs must be very gently eased toward the stirrups. Using a wheelchair and having the help of an attendant, Jack can do little physically on his own. Yet when he mounts his horse, he becomes a different man. Within minutes his body begins to lose its tension, his legs extend, and he sits up high on the saddle, looking for all the world like a jockey, with a certain finesse to his relationship with his horse.

Bill is an attorney who suffered a stroke and some paralysis. He is all business, handles his horse, Cocoa, with authority, and needs very little help. He is the most advanced rider and seems eager to improve his skills. And Andy is a child of maybe seven, darling, wide-eyed, who comes (with one of his parents) because he has learning disabilities, may be hyperactive. He was frightened when he started, didn't want his parents to leave his side, clung to them. But he is a boy positively blossoming on his horse. After a few weeks he was itching for more games in the ring, exercises, competition.

Now he practically ignores his father or mother, has eyes and ears only for his pony, Pepper, and for Lisl, the instructor. Healthy independence seems to be developing.

Lisl Hislop, warm, full of good humor, down to earth, genuine, runs her own horse farm near Palmer, Massachusetts, and as far as I can see participates in the therapeutic riding program as a labor of love. She has long drives back and forth, and whatever she is paid could not be enough. Lisl sees what every rider needs, giving each one the individual attention necessary for something to happen on the ride. And that is the key: something *does* happen when the riders mount their horses. Tight muscles loosen, loose muscles tighten, as human comes in sync with animal. A new rhythm is established, that of two bodies working together, and it seems to have healing properties. I asked Lisl about it once, and she said a horse's gait is similar to that of the human walking. All the same parts of the body are exercised on horseback as would be walking (and the three adults who come don't walk easily or at all). The horse must also give a sense of agency to someone who can't do certain things for himself; it must allow the rider to feel himself in a position of control with his body that might not ordinarily be available to him.

The horses are an integral part of the healing equation, for they are sharing their own horsey vitality with the human atop them, giving of themselves: gentle, mostly patient (sometimes less so), willing to take on unbalanced weight, their healthy muscled bodies, their warmth, their smells all contributing something alive and quivering and sentient. What heals, I sense, is just being on the horse, connecting, one body embracing another in a very physical way, so that all the life that is in the horse can be shared by the rider. A horse can fill a body with life in a kind of pure vitality, concentrated to its essence like homeopathic medicine. A direct hit of life, conveyed body to body, skin to skin, muscle to muscle, is administered in this program.

Lisl has seen remarkable improvements in people in the program over the years. Paralyzed limbs may not be restored, but the riders become bigger people, willing to take risks, open, enthusiastic: more whole. Anytime life opens up this way, a measure of healing has taken place. Anytime something cramped relaxes, whether it is a muscle, a memory, or an attitude, that is healing. Anytime something hard can be transformed into softness, that is healing. Anytime we can join with another living being in mutuality, that is healing. Connection, rhythm, life touching life—these are ways of partaking of what is available to us in the world in which we are enmeshed, the living world, composed of things bright and beautiful, like horses, extraordinary creatures that they are. They hold something healing for us, just as we hold something for the nonhuman world. Appropriate relation, it might be called. When we discover ways to live in appropriate relation, we all benefit. Small joinings, there in the ring at Mount Holyoke's stables, nothing dramatic, but making big differences for everyone involved, healing differences.

weekly gentleness

The Northampton Yoga Center sits on the third floor of a funky old turn-of-the-century Roman revival–style office building on Main Street called the Fitzwilly Building; a point of renown about it is that Calvin Coolidge used to have a law office there. Upon entering, you have a choice in ascending: the gracious, wide staircase, its wooden banister worn to a fine sheen by generations of hands sliding up and down it, or the elevator, an old caged Otis contraption decorated with wrought iron, stained glass, and carved wood; it's due to be renovated before long and should be an even greater delight when restored. The elevator is operated by a small woman with a wizened face who has made the elevator (which holds three people, max) into her own little den, a home away from home. It's filled with pillows, clock, radio, fan, her lunch box, books, magazines, and other assorted stuff, altogether a cozy affair. I have no doubt she could hunker down there for quite a while if necessary.

On the third floor, at the back of a series of mazelike hallways, is the Yoga Center, housed in a room so beautiful that it takes your breath away upon entering. Once used by Masons for fraternal purposes, it is a vast room with ceilings two stories high. Gold molding in a Corinthian motif runs around the top of the walls, with floor-to-ceiling plaster columns repeated every several yards. The walls are painted a serene off-white, but the room is somewhat dark because there are only two (albeit large) windows facing the street. The carpeting is sea-green, punctuated by the colors of the yoga mats, bolsters, straps, and such used in the classes, which are deep purple, mauve, aqua, and ivory. The spaciousness, its colors and pro-portions, is a gift. It is unusual to find clean, pure, pleasing space where you can go and feel there is plenty for everyone! Merely to walk into this room is restorative—your mind and spirit are invigorated and quieted at the same time, swept up in the grandness of it, yet also in the sense of calm.

Before landing here, I had tried for two or three years to find a yoga class I liked, but they had always felt too strenu-ous to me. My friend Thea kept encouraging me to look around, saying a good teacher would make all the difference. One day I saw a flyer for a yoga class for people with arthri-tis and other joint problems. It promised that the class was gentle and easy. I had been having some back problems, so thought it might help. I called, showed up, stepped into that room, met the teacher, Lucy, and knew I had discovered a source of healing.

Lucy used to be a dancer, but she got sick and, she told the class, was unable to do much of anything physical for a year except go to a yoga class and return immediately to bed. Yoga helped heal Lucy, and she was so passionate about it that she trained to teach it. In her leotard and leggings, she still looks every bit the dancer, trim and muscled and able to move and hold her body in beautiful postures. She has a small frame, long, curly hair, and a hypnotic voice that she uses to good ef-fect in the class: I once slept through more than forty-five minutes of class, so deeply relaxing were Lucy's instructions (those instructions were not to sleep, however). What is most striking about her, though, is the quality of her gentleness, which shows on her face, in her movements, in everything about her: a defining characteristic, absolutely embodied.

Lucy is mindful of the variety of physical problems among the people in the class, and she helps each person find what is comfortable and works for him or her. Her message is that most of us tend to push ourselves too hard in life, and in this class, we do not push. Not only do we not push, but we are gentled by Lucy's thoughtful, tender, and caring approach and touch. She reiterates her prophetic word in different ways, several times each session, week after week. Don't push. Go easy on yourself. Extend your limits a bit, then relax. Go slowly. Breathe into the muscles as they work. Stretch, but don't overexert. And always there are her kind voice and her gentle, merciful attitude behind her words, embodying them. I can remember nowhere else I have ever been told to be gentle with myself, to honor pain, to do things slowly, easily, loosely. The messages I have been given (along with many people, I assume) told me to push myself as hard as I could, to go *faster* rather than slower, to have "drive," to "work hard, play hard." Lucy tells us that the opposite is true if we are to grow more healthy. She tells us not to try hard. She urges us to pace ourselves, to work in accord with our rhythms, to treat ourselves gently. Pain should be attended to, not masked so that we can go on working.

In a culture obsessed with striving to get ahead, to succeed, to triumph, it is healing to hear a counter voice urging me to let up, let go, relax, breathe instead of clench. It is healing to put my body into "restorative poses" that help me to relax, utterly. Yoga is helping my flexibility, my body, but Lucy heals the soul by applying a balm of her own. To be touched with extreme gentleness, to feel the quality of mercy, which is, indeed, not strained: the entire being responds because we are soft animals and we need softness to keep supple, healthy, and whole. It is part of who we are, but such a neglected part! Lucy touches the neglected parts and restores something vital. It is healing to be dosed with gentleness weekly just because it is so lacking in our taut, sinewy lives. Not easy to find, perhaps, but nonetheless out there, tucked away here and there, a true gift needing to be received. For Lucy to be able to give her gifts, there must be people to receive them. It's a truth, which is what makes me certain that such merciful moments are available in ordinary days, for the claiming—though perhaps not without some seeking. One year or two spent searching for the right teacher seemed to be a long time, but the effort was well rewarded: beauty, peace, and merciful gentleness once a week, prescription for healing.

· 18 ·

quaker meeting

The Florida Avenue Friends Meeting House in Washington, D.C., is a beautiful fieldstone building that sits back from the street a bit, surrounded by a wrought iron fence and simple yard that blooms with glorious azaleas in spring. I used to park nearby when going to a favorite Indian restaurant at DuPont Circle, but the thought never entered my mind to actually enter it until after my younger brother died in 1980. Some months after his death I walked by once again, this time on a Sunday morning, and it was as if I was actually pulled inside: I could not resist the force that seemed to be dragging me in. It can be difficult to enter the sacred place of a tradition you don't know, and I entered with some trepidation. As soon as I set foot in the simple meeting room inside, however, I felt at home in a profound way. I took a seat, joined in the silence, and my body and soul lapped up the quiet like someone dying of thirst who encounters a pure, fresh stream of water. Pure and fresh were precisely what it was, the enveloping mantle of gathered folks coming together in silence.

It was warm; some people fanned themselves with the rush fans provided, and the slight swish of air being moved gave a cadence to the silence. I sank farther into the peace: my mind quieted; my breath became less shallow; I opened to God, whose presence I felt there among the group. People did talk—the Florida Avenue meeting is known as a chatty one because of the tourists and protesters who so often attend while in the capital city—but I was able to maintain a sense of quiet. I listened with one ear to those inspired to speak. (At a Quaker meeting, people listen to God within, speaking out what comes to them, with discernment, generally. There should be sufficient time in between to take in what has been given voice. It is egalitarian—no one really leads the service, though persons are designated to end the meeting or respond to any unruly worshipers.) And with the other ear I listened to the growing quiet I felt within me. It was something entirely different from any type of worship I had previously known, and it felt true and genuine. It was just what I needed at that time, when I was searching for ways to heal from my brother's death at his own hand. I had put much effort into recovering, but this coming into silence was effortless. Giving myself over to silence was, I see now, giving myself over to God, who did indeed commence to heal me, once I stopped my own frantic efforts.

Silence is a "place" to meet God. We need infusions of quiet to recalibrate ourselves somehow, or let God do the work of calibration. Is it possible that each of us carries within us some memory, or a remnant, of the silence of our Source, somewhat like we carry the little bit left of our tails in our lower backs? Something that stretches *way* back to a time before language? If indeed there is something left within us that recalls the original silence and responds so powerfully, then the moments when we are able to recall it would have a healing effect, calling us back to the "place just right," to where we are plumb with God.

People go to nature to find quiet: fly-fishing, hiking, snowshoeing, walking, or cross-country skiing. People pay top dollar for quiet in noisy places like New York City, where the priciest restaurants are also the most subdued. People respond to the hush of sacred places, whether it is a grove of redwood trees or the nave of a great cathedral. People seek quiet spots in the country for vacations, and there is a boom in people seeking to stay in retreat houses run by religious orders, some of which enforce a rule of silence. As the world grows noisier, filled with relentless communication by cell phone, CD-ROM, Walkman, Watchman, the search for quiet seems to increase proportionately. And though quiet may be hard to come by in some places, the determined seeker can usually find it somewhere for a few moments.

Quiet heals. As far back as the ancient Greeks, people were treated with quiet at the temples of Asclepius, the Greek god of healing, where the ill would be ushered into inner rooms to lie on couches and rest, so that Asclepius might come to them in dreams. In more recent times, quiet was a feature of sanatoriums and hospitals. The effects of quiet may be physiological, a way to give the nervous system a break from constant stimulation; it may be spiritual, providing an interior sanctuary within which one can open herself to God; it may be a way to rest the mind, in order to think clearly, like Thoreau, who sought solitude in the woods in order to reflect and write. It may be any of that, or none of it, but it is a need we have. Finding quiet when it is needed can feel like salvation, restoring our bearings, bringing us back into alignment with life as it was meant to be, reflective of God. In extraordinary moments, in just the time and place when it is sorely needed, quiet can heal, quiet found in ordinary days, ordinary ways.

· 19 ·

trust is not optional

In the spring of 1995 my partner's son, and only child, Chris, then twenty-five years old, tall, attractive, athletic, flew home from California, where he was studying graphic design at the California College of Arts and Crafts, having been told he had cancer. (The first misdiagnosis had been Kaposi's sarcoma; that was changed to some other undefined, rare, fast-growing, deadly sarcoma.) His father, mother, and I took him immediately to the Dana-Farber Institute in Boston, where yet another biopsy was conducted. After days of waiting, word finally came back: Hodgkin's disease. We practically celebrated! Hodgkin's has a high cure rate, and after the emotional seesaw Chris had been on the past weeks, it seemed practically benign by comparison to the other possibilities he had mistakenly, and cruelly, been told.

Once the disease was diagnosed, his doctors drew up a course of treatment with Chris that included chemotherapy every other week for six months, followed by radiation. That was the medical approach. His mother and I mapped out our own, intuitive one. We figured that when life is weakened or threatened, it stands to reason that life must be stimulated and strengthened in response. We tried to do everything we could to create an environment where life would be catalyzed toward healing. It took some work, and a lot of trust in ourselves, to marshal all available energy in the service of Chris's survival.

We moved a comfortable chair and stool out onto our porch, which is open on three sides to the garden that surrounds it, so that Chris could sit or doze within sight and smell of ripening fruit trees, fragrant old roses and herbs, fresh new grasses and hay from the open fields beyond the house. We placed the bird feeder so that birds could be seen from his chair, not more than ten feet away, and filled it with thistle seed to tempt the bright yellow goldfinches to stay close, along with the downy woodpeckers, chickadees, and cardinals. Ensconced thus, Chris spent hours on the porch, taking in the life that enveloped him.

Then we made a list of people, friends of Chris and friends of ours, whom we considered full of life, fun, good listeners, or good talkers, most of all good laughers (à la Norman Cousins). We invited them to visit from around the country, around the world, and a steady stream of visitors came and went all summer. On that porch we drank cold Sam Adams beer and ate lots of good, fresh foods (grilled salmon with ginger-lime-cilantro salsa, tender, fresh, young greens in salads, ripe peaches and melons, crusty, chewy bread, poached eggs from local hens kept by a woman called Chicken Carol), sitting for hours at the round glass table, talking and laughing. Rachel, Jane Ann, Thea, John and Mary (from County Cork, Ireland, bearing especially raucous laughter and prize-winning stories!), Treva, Mark, Margaret, Lou and Read, Tom: they brought healing medicine; they brought themselves. All joined in, consciously or unconsciously, to lift Chris up, and lift they did. The guests supported life by being, not doing, but it was work. To promote life in this way, to keep the juices flowing, to keep the air crackling with good energy, takes a lot. It takes an outpouring of vitality and presence, the willingness to extend one's life force on behalf of another, and the ability to be open and stand with someone facing death. It takes trust in Being itself.

Summer turned into fall, the guests tapered off, the porch was closed up for winter, chemotherapy was replaced by radiation, the tumor shrank, and finally, by New Year's Eve 1996, the treatment was over, the cancer gone. To then recover from the experience of *fighting* cancer took enormous energy itself—we were all so focused on the struggle that when it was over, we were completely spent. Chris was depressed to be living at home again at age twenty-five, trying to get enough money together to get back into school and move out (but to Boston, not California, because he had to remain close to Dana-Farber for periodic checkups over the next few years). He was able to do so by the following May, graduating in 1998 from the Massachusetts College of Art, having received the Outstanding Senior award for his work there. He had successfully traversed a dangerous passage and moved on.

Chris is an extremely thoughtful man, keenly observant, sensitive, intuitive, someone who has always seemed much older than whatever age he was because of his understanding and wisdom: an old soul. The experience with illness deepened him even more, having moved him into a place that young people don't usually have to go. (I remember a conversation with him toward the end of the treatment when he said he felt out of place at parties, how he could no longer happily just drink beer and carouse, because it seemed so superficial.) He lost his youth abruptly, being forced to deal with his own death head-on. But with some time and distance, he was able to integrate the experience and derive meaning from it that is and will be an essential part of his life to come. After we had all recovered from the experience of cancer, I sat down with Chris to ask him what *he* believed had helped to heal him.

Chris named some particulars that helped in the healing, starting with the fact that upon his arrival home from

California, his best friend Sean's father, Dr. Joe Kelly, came over immediately to examine him and serve as his primary care physician so that he might be officially referred to Dana-Farber. That made him feel safe. He believed that Joe cared about what happened to him, and he therefore trusted him to act in his best interests, unlike the erstwhile doctor he had seen in San Francisco.

At Dana-Farber Chris was assigned to a youngish doctor whom he connected with. He felt "seen" by this doctor; he didn't feel like "just another" Hodgkin's case. But then, Chris did everything he could to make sure he *was* seen for who he was. He says he did everything he could to be a "good patient" to elicit attention by being informed, upbeat, bright, witty. When the stakes are survival, you do whatever you can to bring the medical establishment's attention to bear on you (that our medical system *requires* such strategies from those who are ill is disgraceful). Nonetheless, the doctor-patient pairing developed into a relationship based on trust. The nurse who actually delivered his chemo by infusion was another person Chris trusted completely. If she had slipped up in any way, delivering too heavy a dose of toxins into his system, it could have killed him. Chris felt her confidence from the beginning, which inspired his own confidence and trust. Because he could trust her, he did not waste any of his precious energy being anxious about the treatment itself.

Family and friends were also important. Chris distinguished between those who were able to give love, attention, and concern, those he could trust to be there for him, and those who couldn't, and he tried to avoid the ones who couldn't. Illness can bring a variety of people into one's life, and just because they appear on the scene doesn't mean the one who is ill needs to receive them. With his keen sense of what *he* needed to do to survive, Chris cut quickly (and precisely) to essentials and spent no more time than absolutely necessary with anyone who drained him. The people who *were* there included Mark, a poet friend who knew how to listen; Sean and his medical school friends, with whom Chris felt safe to hang out, trusting they wouldn't "freak" if something happened to him; Rachel, a fabulous-looking woman who flirted with him over one weekend, bearing the vitality of sexual attraction; his immediate family, who marshaled every possible resource to help him through; and family friends who supported Chris by supporting us all.

And then there was Chris himself, his own best possible physician. From the very beginning of the journey, he knew he would be fine, even if he died. He came in touch with his core self, some truth that was his alone. Coming to know that part of himself, Chris says, enabled him to totally trust *himself*. Not arrogantly, because he had certainly been humbled, but confidently, and with steely determination. He knew within himself what he had to do to get better, and he trusted that because it came from the very deepest part of his being. He knew from this place that he had to keep an open mind, for instance, so that he was willing to try almost anything, talk with anyone, reach out in ways he had not before. (One thing he learned by accident that seemed to help him quite a bit, and he then stuck by for the entire course of chemotherapy, was stopping at McDonald's for lunch before a chemo treatment. Later that day and evening he felt much better, and less nauseated, than on any previous treatment day. Chris's theory is that the high fat content of the food may have absorbed the harsh toxins, acting as a kind of sponge to his system. He ate at McDonald's on every chemo trip thereafter and still swears by it!) Although Chris would not describe himself as a religious person, he welcomed the prayers that his mother and I solicited from anyone, everywhere we went. We had individuals and groups praying for him around the world. (Chris's last name is Reese. Someone in our home church who didn't know Chris thought that we were praying every week for Christopher Reeve, the actor who had been paralyzed not long before, so she spent six months praying for him instead. We assume it helped him!)

These aspects of his recovery are part of Chris's story and may or may not pertain to healing more generally. What strikes me about his account of his journey is the emphasis on trust and what it meant to him. Without trust, according to Chris, you can't focus your energy on getting well: it gets siphoned off into fear and anxiety. He is saying, I think, that trust is a given that *must* be there. It is not optional. Trust from various sources "coalesced into power," to use Chris's words, a vital source to be called upon in the work of healing. In seeking healing, we must marshal all the possible sources of trust we are able to, and diminish, as much as possible, the role of those who are not trustworthy. We all have pretty good ideas of the people we trust and the people we don't, the people we know from ordinary places such as the neighborhood, work, church, school, clubs. We must learn to trust ourselves enough to listen to our own instincts and move away from people or places where we are not supported. By a combination of confidence, intuition, and common sense, Chris called into his life every bit of trust that he could, and it helped heal him. Trust is available to all of us in everyday life, in varying degrees. We can cultivate it, as Chris did, and it can help heal us too.

· 20 ·

sunday school revisited

After my younger brother died in 1980, I realized I needed help coping with his death. I knew one or two people in therapy at that time, and I asked one of them for the name of her therapist: Barbara Hammer. I began seeing Barbara, worked through, as best as I could, my grief for my brother, dealt with some additional issues, and in due time was ready to finish therapy. In a discussion one day in which I told Barbara I felt ready to leave, she told me she thought there were two areas I had not yet addressed: smoking and God! I had never thought of either of them as concerns for psychotherapy, but I was anxious to finish up, and so told Barbara I would stop smoking within a month, which I did. But God was another matter!

I asked Barbara what she thought I needed to "do" about God. She said that she had never heard me mention God, that I seemed to have no spiritual life, and that perhaps that was something I needed. We had never discussed God or anything remotely religious in my family, even though we had attended church weekly. I was embarrassed to talk about this subject with Barbara, much more embarrassed than I was when talking about sexual matters. Certainly it *was* true that I needed to "deal with" God.

Barbara asked me whether I believed in God. I said no, I did not, because I just could not accept the idea that there was a big old man with a white beard somewhere, sitting ready to judge us. She asked, What made me think that was God? I replied because "they" said so, "everyone" said so. Who? she asked. Oh, my Sunday school teachers and, I supposed, the pope. So what made me think (if indeed this was the case) that they were right? I was astonished at Barbara's questioning the authority of the pope! I was a Protestant, but grew up in a Catholic neighborhood. I had ceded as much authority to the pope as any good Catholic child did. In the realm of religion, his presumed views were definitive for me.

Barbara pressed on. No one, as far as she knew, had ever seen God and reported back. And no living person could know any more about God than any other person since it all came down to speculation in the end. Some, it is true, were trained in theology, spiritual practices, and the like, but that still didn't mean they necessarily knew any more than anyone else did. In the field of theology, there are no irrefutable "proofs." (Trying to recall this conversation, I am aware that I am probably simplifying it terribly now: I don't claim these to be Barbara's exact words, but how I heard them, what they meant to me.) And in that case, my idea of God would be as valid as anyone else's.

Why didn't I try to think about an image of God that made sense to me now, something I *could* believe in? I think she must also have pointed out that my concept was that of a seven- or eight-year-old, that I seemed to have gotten stuck somewhere back in a Sunday school class and never progressed beyond it in terms of my faith development. That was true, and I have since learned that it happens to others, too, especially those who were given a picture of God by some strong authority. Left with such an untenable God image, we think that our only recourse is complete rejection. All of this, the very idea of reworking the image I had been given, the idea that I might come up with my own way of relating to

God, made me feel that I had just come upon the burning bush, so revealing was it for me! (Neither Barbara nor I am saying one's personal image of God *is* God. But it is a doorway to a *belief* in God.)

Barbara didn't stop there, however. For the first and only time since I had been seeing her, she asked me to lie down on her couch, and when I did, she led me through a guided meditation calling on God's healing power. I felt that power come into me, work through me, and when the time on the couch was over, I *was* healed of a serious wound: at age thirty-four, I was finally able to believe in God. Barbara had acted as a healer in a capacity far beyond that of therapist, delivering me back to God so that God might work in me and eventually through me. It was pure grace at work, her bringing this up at precisely the right moment, a moment at which I could take it in. In the most profound sense, she, an agent of healing, moved me into greater wholeness, the wholeness available to us when our lives are centered on God. Although it was just the first small step toward such a recentering, it was, for me, a life-defining moment, the moment I was turned toward my true center. I had no idea that day when I drove up Rock Creek Parkway that my life would be changed. A healing touch can await us like that, anytime, anyplace. It was just an ordinary day. Or so I thought.

· 21 ·

in the garden

Gardening has become big business in the United States over the past dozen years or so. Marketing experts say the reason is that baby boomers, who are now middle-aged and have raised their children, have time and disposable income on their hands. Maybe so, but I believe that people are sinking their hands into earth for another reason: because it heals. In some twenty-five years of gardening, I've learned a few things, and one thing I know is that being outside connected to earth and air and sun can bring a person into intimate connection with the created world, and apprehending one's place in the creation has the capacity to heal.

A garden is a work in process, as any gardener knows, a life project that is never finished until one dies. It reflects its laborer, who is also a work in process. As we grow and are inspired to change, so do our gardens. A stand of Siberian iris that seemed absolutely perfect when put in wants digging out three years later; raspberry bushes that were just the thing seem to turn overnight into unruly characters menacing anything close to their ever-expanding borders; orange daylilies no longer suffice against a fence, for something more subtle is needed. Our tastes change and our garden visions are constantly being remade by what we see, read, dream up. Five years come and go, and the five-year plan needs changing.

Life is process, constantly changing us, constantly requiring us to change. In some areas of life—work, relationships—

we can hold out longer, dance around, avoid or prolong changing. But the garden shows us inescapably that it and we are *always* in transition, and it had best not be fought. In the garden we cannot avoid accepting the constancy of change. There we live with it, do what must be done, with far less of the grousing and stalling than we do in other places of our lives because we come fairly quickly to see that grousing in the garden is futile. It does not respond. It is not in our control. It is a constant—constant change—to which we must adjust.

Once we learn this basic lesson and change ourselves to work *with* it rather than trying to squeeze it into the form we had in mind, the garden begins to really come alive, to find its own best form. For years I selected perennials from glossy catalogs, lusting after certain color schemes, height, effect. Slowly, it dawned on me to work with what is local, tried, and true: the classics of New England gardens. The oddities have been replaced (those that didn't die out of their own accord) with local standards: lilacs, peonies, purple coneflowers, asters, phlox, bee balm. The garden shaped itself. I followed. So too, when we learn to accept life as it presents itself, working with it rather than trying to impose our own determined wills on it, *we* come alive. Resistance, struggle, stress—they all come from fighting something alien to us that we have planted in our psychic gardens rather than finding what suits us best and moving with it. Clenching in resistance is not a healthy way to live. Accepting and moving with change, rather than being moved by our own self-determined effort, is.

And then there are the seasons of the garden, and the wait for the perfect moment when it is at its peak, the moment we invite guests to see. Pruned and trimmed and ready, party planned, and a week of rain wipes out the lilacs and the peonies, nothing to show, and the party must be held inside a damp house, lamps lit against the dark downpour. We learn our garden lessons season by season by season, over and over and over: out there, we must live in the moment, for it is only the moment we ever have in a garden. We want to plan ahead, we order six climbing roses for the splendid vision we have in mind, but winter kills, moths eat, moles tunnel, fruit drops, and we learn to settle for what *is* at any given time. The harsh conditions set down by nature may annoy, may drive us to utter frustration, yet I have never heard of someone giving up on gardening (unless because of bad back or ill health) the way I've heard of someone throwing his golf clubs into a lake after an especially bad round, never to play again. A fledgling gardener will struggle some with this reality, but eventually acceptance does set in, and acceptance of life's conditions is healing in that the body/mind/spirit has the opportunity to come into alignment with truth. If we can flow along with it, moment by moment, wherever it takes us, we are likely to become more whole.

In a garden we can come to feel our place in the created world, seeing how it all works together, and seeing that our part has very little to do with any results that may happen. The world was made not just for us humans, but for every living creature that also calls it home. The idea of dominion dies off for anyone spending much time in a garden because one quickly learns that she does not, indeed, *have* dominion. A gardener may plant the seed, work the earth, prune the trees, do any of the endless chores that await her there, but what *cause* the seed to grow, the bush to fruit, are water and sun and fertile earth and the mysterious forces of growth. Too much wind, sun, or water; earth leached of nutrients; too little water or warmth; severe winter, warm winter; any and all of the interferences that can come from nature can wreak havoc with the best efforts of the best gardener. Moles, raccoons, deer, Japanese beetles, gypsy moths, worms, bugs, birds—everything must be perfectly balanced in the chain of life for it to work, and as we have sadly learned, extinction of any species may throw the balance off and cause serious repercussions. All of this is going on in the garden all the time, and any gardener who spends some time paying attention, observing, will soon enough know that her place is but a small one in the entire scheme.

How does this knowledge heal? By coming into right relationship with the rest of nature, we discover that we are responsible only for our own little acre. It's an example of living locally, thinking globally. We must till our plot, do all we can to make it flourish, while leaving the larger scheme in God's hands.

You can do only what you can do. This is not, of course, an excuse to avoid doing all that you can to improve life for others, in whatever ways you can. But knowing that you are but one small unit of the entire scheme of life, you cultivate your garden as best you can and know that whatever comes out of it is not up to you alone. Accepting change, living in the moment, knowing your place in the creation: three truths gleaned in the garden, healing truths if you can learn to live by them.

· 22 ·

simple basics

Anyone who keeps an eye on gardening equipment may have seen, in the past few years, terra-cotta pots covered with multicolored shards of pottery, tiles, and dishes. The potter and tile maker Susan Parks designed such pots as a way to recycle all the broken tiles she has amassed over the years. Creating a beautiful object out of waste is the kind of thing Susan is wont to do. In her life, there is little waste of any kind, having stripped her wants and needs down to the simple basics. Susan is an artist (and spent fifteen years as a tenured professor of art before leaving it behind to make and sell tiles), so she is creative, and she is also practical, good with her hands in a Yankee kind of way, able to piece together a chicken coop from scrap lumber, at home chopping wood and carrying water when on retreat in the woods meditating, a superb cook who works attentively in the kitchen with the perfect ingredients she has chosen. Her small home is spare and uncluttered; she keeps at hand only what she needs, and her needs are few. Whatever *is* in her life is apt to be carefully chosen, aesthetically pleasing, and useful. A clean room, a few beautifully glazed mugs, a wildflower or two on the table, a small, perfect garden, a place to work clay, a lamb or two, a few chickens: Susan's life is well defined, precise, and lean, yet abundantly rich. Rich with experience, rich with time, available to her to use as she will because she pursues only what she values, only what works for her.

In her fifties, a woman with a perpetual trace of a smile and lively, sparkling eyes, Susan has a hint of a pixie about her, almost fey. She is fun, extremely witty, a gracious guest, and a generous host. She likes to play and knows how to bring others into the world of play with her. There is no heaviness to her, and time spent with Susan is always rejuvenating. She was not always so buoyant of spirit, however. She spent a number of years struggling as she sought to go her own way, to shape her life as carefully as she shapes clay. To come to this state of rich leanness, Susan had to go through a series of givings up: a good job with a dependable and comfortable income, an identity handed to her by family and culture, desires and fears large and small, people who drained her, and more, as much as she could strip off to let the authentic Susan emerge.

For the past fifteen years or so she has practiced Zen Buddhism. By this point, after years of practicing clearing her mind of its "monkeys," she has cleared so much extraneous matter out of her self that she is able to be present to others in ways rarely seen in anyone devoting less effort. What is particular to Susan's presence is that, because she has done so much work to develop consciousness and because she realizes that each person has a path and process of his or her own, she has the capacity to be with people while letting them be and not obstructing their paths in any way. To be with, yet not obstruct: compassion that seems to stem from her experience as a Buddhist, but embodied in Susan's own, particular way. She has learned that "making better" is often not the most helpful position when it comes to people struggling with life issues; rather, *not* shielding them from confronting their own issues is the compassionate way (though certainly the much more difficult one). Allowing people to take the consequences of their own actions is the only way they can learn what they're doing. If you jump in to fix, says Susan, you are intruding with your agenda for them, how you think things "ought" to be. You are assuming you know what is best for someone else. To not obstruct takes much greater courage. To not do is healing. How is this so?

Anyone who knows Susan Parks loves being with her, running into her for a few minutes on the street when she comes to town to do errands, driving the big old Checker cab that serves as her car, her border collie in the passenger seat, or spending a few hours with her sharing a good meal (rare, because she takes care to spend her energy wisely). Being in her presence feels good because she is clear about who *she* is and who *you* are, and she pays enormous attention to you without ever imposing her own agenda, without judging, without manipulating. If you went to Susan with a problem, you could be sure she would not give advice, console, intrude. She would be wholly present and conscious of what she was *not* doing. She would care if you were in pain, and that would be evident to you, for her caring is all the more intense because not clouded by her own pain, her own struggles. She would hold herself back, and that is what feels so restoring: caring attention without a stake in the outcome. (This could be called unconditional love, but that would not be Susan's way of describing it, I don't imagine. She would make it more understandable.) Being joined by someone who understands where you are without entering into where you are can lessen anxiety and fear. Anytime you can let go of fear, you receive a portion of healing, for fear binds you to something less than fullness. Fear sets up dualities ("you" against "them"), binds to brokenness. And to know someone else can face what you perhaps cannot gives hope, hope that you will somehow be able to walk down a similar path, clear yourself of your own fears. If one person has done so, others can.

To rub up against someone like Susan is healing because she so *embodies* in her daily, ordinary self all that she has brought to bear so that she might live out of an authentic center. An encounter with Susan is never a "head trip." She is always there with you, present and accounted for. Her Buddhism, her experience, her wisdom—all is concrete, real, and available. It's not a belief system she adheres to, but beliefs-in-the-process of being realized in the world (or practice). She heals through her way of being in the world, which is absolutely concrete. There is nothing abstract about Susan, though she is extremely intelligent, witty, original, articulate. In fact, she can articulate abstractions better than anyone I know: she can make something extremely complex understandable, and in this way is a teacher as well as a healer. Just as she has simplified her life in a complex world, Susan simplifies all kinds of heady ideas, puts flesh on them so that you can get a grasp on their essence. She can do this because she knows what is essential and what is not. When my partner, Nancy, and I were preparing to move to New York City, Susan came over for a goodbye lunch and threw out a few simple words about New York and money. She told us to prepare to have money flow out all the time there, that New York was all about the exchange of money, and it was best to see that and accept it, so we wouldn't be anxious all the time over cost and how much we were spending, compared to how little we made there. Just let it flow, said Susan, you cannot expect to hold onto money in New York. It will come back at some other time. She was right, of course, and being able to part easily with our small stores of money helped make bearable what could have been a terrible burden. It was a modern version of the lilies-of-the-field parable: don't be anxious about how you will get along; you will be fine. Indeed!

Making important concepts understandable to common folk, translating her observations into concrete details, conveying a sense of solidity and "hereness," all anchor whoever

Susan is with, and the anchoring is life affirming, health giving. That anchoring counters fear, balances all the clattering, nattering thoughts and voices in your head, helps siphon off some of the stuff that obstructs your own life force. Susan frees up what is in you to flow as it should, removing barriers, unclogging what has been stopped up, setting you free because she is free, or at least showing you it is possible. It is her gift, her art, her practice, her life, all of a piece.

When one person moves toward wholeness, it shows we all can, and that is the essence of healing: moving toward wholeness. Susan is truly a physician who has healed herself and now heals others. Look for her, or others of her ilk, at the lumberyard, veterinarian's clinic, hardware store: ordinary places.

23

out of time

My maternal grandmother, Constance Palmer, whom we called Nana, was a part of our family (four children, two parents) from the time my older sister, Sue, the first child, was born until Nana died in her eighties. Our house was a large one, and Nana had her own quarters in the back of the house, a spacious room with windows on three sides and bookshelves lining the remaining wall space. There was a little gas-powered fireplace in the corner, and facing it were her couch and a rocking chair. The bookshelves were a necessity, for Nana was a scholar with a voracious appetite for books. She was unusual in her time, a woman who had gone to college before the turn of the century and then taught Latin and Greek before marrying and bearing eight children in thirteen years. Living with us, she made bread every week, baby-sat, mended, did a variety of other chores, and spent the rest of her time reading and writing. Once a week she would take the bus downtown to the main branch of the Cleveland Public Library and come home bearing brown paper sacks of books for herself, for my mother, and for us children. Almost every evening, the incentive for my sister and me to bathe and get ready for bed was that we would be read to. In her cozy space we'd snuggle next to Nana on the couch, covered with an afghan, and there be transported into the world of fairy tale and story. In winter, she'd make tea and toast in the little kitchen station set up in a corner of her bathroom. Later, as we grew older, my sister would sometimes join her in late night sessions, watching Jack Paar on television together from the same couch.

Nana was from Virginia, and she had a soft, southern-accented voice. She was, above all, a gentle woman, and being with her was gentling, soothing, easy. She demanded nothing, luring us instead into her world, where poetry, in English and in Latin, was recited by heart even when she later began to lose her memory for what was happening in the here and now; where fairy tales came alive with her reading, into which she put much energy; where my first childhood goal that I can remember (inspired, of course, by Nana) was applying for my own library card (whenever I could sign my name). Reading, writing, and learning were inextricably entwined with Nana's softness, her welcoming coziness, her patience, her love for us. And she was this way with everyone. This is not merely a grandchild's memory, for neighborhood children would come by to see and be tutored by her and adults loved to visit with her.

What I believe she offered people was respite from all the busyness of life, even a child's life. Nana was a living, walking oasis for all who encountered her. Never in a hurry, slow, gentle and kind, patient and modest, she was *inviting,* and once you accepted the invitation and came into the circle of her influence, she transported you to a different world, the world of literature, poetry, story, tall tales, doggerel: pure rhyme, fantasy, magic, a world where anything was possible. She was formed by literature, history, the classics, myth, and all that she had taken in, in a lifetime of reading, had become a part of her being. To be with her was to enter not just into the world of the mind, but something much more, a world where eternal verities were real, where beauty and truth reigned supreme, where good triumphed over evil, maidens were rescued, frogs became princes, fairies sewed suits of clothes for tailors overnight.

Nana *lived* in that place, not in any way as an escapist, but as someone who knew the contours and edges of daily life needed smoothing. Having a mind and soul so filled with riches of these sorts, Nana could cross borders into other realms, the realm of spirit (though not in a religious sense). That spirit imbued her to such an extent that anyone spending an hour or two with her was bound to feel it and, if open to it, to be transported there with her. She knew that restorative world well, and since she did, others who encountered her were able to visit there too. Visiting a world of spirit, even so briefly, a world that lies behind, or parallel to, the one we usually live in, gives respite from the stress and struggle and anxieties of the daily world. And respite, temporary relief from pain or travail, gives us the chance to stop and breathe and heal. Stepping out of "time" into a timeless world allows us to exist, momentarily, without the cares and woes of the day. It lightens us, buoys us up.

A moment of respite can heal. It heals by giving us the chance to stop and stand back from where we typically stand in the world; it gives us a way to see things differently from the way that we usually see them. Common wisdom has it that a change of scenery is good for someone who is tired and worn out. Respite of the sort I am talking about is similar, giving a "change of scenery" from the "normal" world, a moment of refreshment. And in such an extraordinary moment, anything can happen, including healing. Vacations may be hard to come by, but the world of literature and tales and poetry is always available, moments to relish in ordinary days.

24

neighbors

Mrs. Pertzoff was my neighbor on East Capitol Street when I lived in Washington, D.C., and worked at the Library of Congress. When I moved in next door to her in the summer of 1976, she took an interest in me because she had retired from the library, where she had worked for years as a shelf lister. A shelf lister assigns the unique number that fits the book into the permanent inventory of the library. Since hundreds of thousands of books flood into the collections of the Library of Congress every year, the job requires meticulous attention. In the good old days, according to Mrs. Pertzoff, the shelf listers wore white cotton gloves to do their work. One fateful day, however, Librarian of Congress Archibald MacLeish called the catalogers and shelf listers together and, standing atop a table in a reading room, implored them to come down from their ivory towers and into the twentieth century. The practice of wearing white gloves was discontinued, a symbol, I suppose, of a new era. Mrs. Pertzoff never quite recovered from the sacrilege, and her retirement was not far behind.

At the time I knew her, Mrs. Pertzoff (her name was Barbara, but I never called her that—too familiar!) and I shared a fence. Our houses, like many of the brick townhouses on our street, had small front gardens, many of which were fenced in with wrought iron, as were ours. We would meet in front, she inspecting her roses, I trying to set a garden growing, and chat. Or more accurately, she talked, I listened.

Mrs. Pertzoff, in her early seventies, was elegant, educated, tended toward haughty, and fussy. She had a vision of how life should be and clung to it tenaciously. She spoke precisely, with impeccable diction, and carried herself with dignity. She was meticulous about her house and garden, and fond of giving me advice on everything from how to tar the roof to the best person to use for window locks. To carry out her own missions, she called upon Henry, her handyman who had worked for her for years and seemed to know just how to respond to her. Though occasionally he did some painting or fixing, his main duty seemed to be to walk over to the liquor store on North Carolina Avenue to pick up Dry Sack sherry and cartons of Merit cigarettes for Mrs. Pertzoff. He was a gentle soul who had passed his prime, but that didn't keep Mrs. Pertzoff and him from having loud, heated arguments from time to time, and then we wouldn't see Henry for a while. Mrs. Pertzoff could be hard to take, as Henry pointed out, and I had little patience for her, especially her long phone calls in the evening telling me what I should do about my house. She was, in short, a trial, despite her gracious side.

As fall moved toward winter, I noted one day that I hadn't seen or heard from Mrs. Pertzoff in a while, and I started to wonder where she was. Eventually, having not laid eyes on Henry for some time, I called upon her, finding her in quite a state. Her house, like mine, had three floors, but she rented her top floor as an apartment and lived on the bottom two, mostly in the basement, which is where I went to find her. The kitchen was in the back; in the front room were wedged a dining room table and chairs for six or eight, chests, a desk, several little tables, an etagère, a couch, all sitting on a gorgeous red Oriental carpet that had belonged to her husband,

Peter. Peter had left Russia as a young man during the revolution, traveling with his brother and mother to Paris, where they settled for a while, and eventually to the United States. (He, too, had worked at the Library of Congress, which is where he and Barbara had met.) Leaving Russia, they had carried gems to sell and some possessions, including the rug. On the walls of this stuffed, now slightly dismal apartment (dismal because unclean and unkempt: huge ashtrays overflowed with cigarette butts because Mrs. Pertzoff was, incongruously, a chain smoker, years of the *New Yorker* sat stacked on the floor and atop the couch where she slept, and there was a distinct doggy smell from her two schnauzers, Hans and Fritz, who lived in the room with her) were paintings by Matisse and Rouault, among others, purchased by Peter during the Paris years.

What I took in among the faded elegance was a woman distressingly ill. She had lost significant weight—she said she had no energy to cook or eat—her eyes looked strange, and her hair was matted, unbrushed in some time. In fact, she seemed to be barely functioning. I was alarmed, suggested I take her to the doctor. It took some pushing to get her to call (and Mrs. Pertzoff was not to be pushed), and it may have taken a few days before she did, but finally we arranged that I would accompany her by taxi since she refused to put me to the trouble of taking her in my car. The doctor, whom I remember well because he was so kind and respectful with her, took one look at her and guessed that her thyroid had gone awry, metabolism screeched to a halt. (Apparently, she had had thyroid problems in the past.) He wanted to put her in the hospital, but she wouldn't hear of that. He asked me if I would be willing to watch over her and my heart sank, but I said I would. He then asked me to feed her as I could, anything to get her weight back up and some strength in her body, and sent her home with a prescription for synthetic thyroid and a diet supplement. Since she was shaky, he also suggested I help her bathe.

I felt that a rather burdensome responsibility had been thrust on me from out of the blue, and I wasn't happy about it. For one thing, Mrs. Pertzoff was persnickety; things had to be just so, and her standards, it seemed, were informed by the imperial Russian court. I had no desire to put myself in line for the criticism Henry inevitably fell heir to. Also, I was worried; her health seemed to have fallen into my twenty-something hands, if only by default. What if she died? It was with real reservations that I accepted the task.

I like to cook, so making meals wasn't difficult. Mrs. Pertzoff didn't like the diet supplement, but she did suggest homemade eggnog, which I made with whipping cream, eggs, and bourbon, a new batch every few days. Every other day I would draw her a bath, help her into it, and wash and dry her, which must have been difficult for her, dignified as she was. It seems to me I found someone to clean the basement. She started to recover quickly once the thyroid got into her system. Christmas was on its way a few weeks after I started helping her, so I invited her to Christmas dinner. I'll never forget her arrival, carrying a purse and a large brown grocery sack, from which, once seated, she withdrew two *cartons* of Merits. That woman could do some smoking! We laughed about the cigarettes together, each softening a bit.

Soon she no longer needed my help, but was ever after grateful, referring to it as "the time you saved my life in '76." Over the next several years, until I moved away in 1985, Mrs. Pertzoff would remark on '76. If indeed I had saved her life, I must admit I did so grudgingly. But before long, I noticed that I began to change in my feelings toward her. She no longer bothered me. In fact, I began to be happy to visit with her and let her regale me with stories, albeit the same ones. Each time, she repeated the mantra: "saved my life in '76." Finally, I grew to love her with a genuine, open-hearted love.

What changed my heart? I opened in response to her attitude toward me; she saw me, rightly or wrongly, as someone who had saved her life and constantly let me know of her gratitude. When someone presents herself with such appreciation, being unresponsive is difficult. In her eyes, I was esteemed, and most of us respond to feeling esteemed. That's no great revelation! What was healing about the encounter, what made those moments—hours—extraordinary, was that in doing something for another, I was made more whole. I grew to be bigger than I had been, stretched by connecting to another being who needed care. We came together purely by circumstance, and out of the circumstances came first respect, then liking, then love.

The healing came not in '76, but later. It came through the love each developed for the other, blossoming out of an ordinary, neighborly encounter. Anytime love enters our lives, it heals. Love carries healing by its very nature. God's love, our love, the love of an animal, whatever form it comes in, love heals. Opening to love in unexpected places, we experience extraordinary moments, and they hold the promise of healing. A somewhat crabby neighbor standing by her fence pointing out paint that is peeling and should be scraped may not appear to be an agent of healing at first glance, but look again—fences come down, cold hearts melt, love happens, and then healing, right next door.

harvesting hope

"Community supported agriculture" is a term used to describe a movement of people seeking to keep small farming viable in the United States. The farmer contracts with a fixed number of people to provide produce for a set fee, five hundred dollars for a "unit" share, for example. (The unit might be established for two adults, but four people might split a unit, depending on how many vegetables they can eat in a week.) Once the growing season begins, those who have contracted for produce pick it up once a week and are given whatever is ready. The buyers get fresh, local, organic produce, and the farmer knows exactly how much money he or she will be paid for the season. By binding themselves together in this way, a large group of people benefit by supporting a local food system, a farmer is able to make a living from agriculture, and the community at large profits from the presence of fertile land in its midst.

Eileen Droescher had long dreamed of owning and operating her own organic farm. As a child, she was raised on a farm where her family grew or raised everything they ate, keeping chickens, sheep, and ducks, growing berries and fruit trees in addition to vegetables. Once she left home she was for several years a teacher, then owned a successful florist and commercial plant business. She built the business up to a point where selling it would give her a grubstake for a piece of land to farm. After a few years on the market, the business finally sold, and Eileen proceeded to apprentice herself over two growing seasons to experienced farmers who taught her what little else she needed to learn in order to pursue her dream.

During the years of selling the business and working on other people's farms, Eileen had also been assiduously looking for her own farm to buy, years during which more and more farmers in our area sold to developers, since there are scant people lined up to buy land to actually farm. The towns around where I live—Southampton, Easthampton, Westhampton—have been farming towns for a few hundred years, but like everywhere else in this country, our towns have grown more and more suburban, less and less rural. Eileen pictured, and prayed for, ten acres and a small, efficient house in the country. Her prayers were eventually answered, but like so many answered prayers, the answer looked a lot different from what she had in mind. An eighteen-acre plot of farmland went on sale in the middle of Easthampton, surrounded on all sides by housing, hardly in the country! The compact house of her vision was instead a large, rambling farmhouse, old and in disrepair. The land, however, was perfect. Considered one of the best farming areas in the lush Connecticut River Valley (itself known for its excellent growing conditions), the soil was classed "One" judged on its composition (mix of sand, clay, silt, rocks, etc.), capacity to hold moisture, and depth of topsoil. Chemicals had not been used on it for many a year. Though nothing like what she had envisioned, it was the place for Eileen.

The property had been inherited and put up for sale by a relative who didn't live in the community, someone who wanted to sell for top dollar, naturally enough. Eileen bid on the property, as did a local developer. The developer kept raising the stakes in order to outbid Eileen. But the town, which had an option on part of the property, called in the Massachusetts Land Conservation Trust to see if they could help: this group helps preserve farms to be worked. Still, the developer kept raising his bid. Soon enough, word got around to the neighbors who lived near the farm that it was likely to be developed, and they raised, incredibly, $80,000 (a significant amount in these parts) to help Eileen, whom none of them knew, get the farm. Other town agencies became involved; the local press covered the story, and quiet, modest, low-profile Eileen became the center of something reaching far beyond her individual efforts to find a farm.

Meanwhile, everyone who knew Eileen was praying hard for her. Finally, Eileen was told that the relative was going to accept the developer's last bid, one that Eileen could not match, even with all the help. In one last attempt to salvage the farm that could be hers, she called the seller and poured out her heart to her, telling her about her dream, how important it is to keep such good soil in farming, how essential land is to the community, all that the property meant to her. The next day, the owner changed her mind and decided to sell to Eileen after all, even though it meant less money for her. Eileen considers it a miracle, as does anyone else who knows all the intricacies of the story!

The closing has come and gone; Eileen now has her dream, and lots of work ahead of her. As mentioned, the dream has a little tarnish to it: two barns in bad repair and full of stuff, literally tons of stuff, along with termite damage and mold. In the house, lots of junk to be sold or carted away, more garbage in the basement, and a long way to go to be livable. But also: house sound, if in need of repairs and much work, architecturally every bit the classic farmhouse; a huge, perfectly shaped maple tree in the yard throwing off a circle of shade that must be forty feet in diameter; and a beautiful piece of land cut through by brooks, sheltered by the base of Mt.

Tom, our local mountain. Eileen is a worker, so she will have the place in top-notch condition as soon as it can be humanly accomplished. She already has plans in place for the winter and spring to begin nourishing the soil. The barn is being renovated. She will do what she has set out to do, with the help of the community and town, now involved in what she had thought was her dream alone. And the rest of us, those who know Eileen and those who don't, will benefit by proxy.

Eileen will restore life to soil that lay fallow. Through her careful tending (and she is a meticulous laborer), her love of the land, and its cultivation, she will give the community a great gift, the gift of germination, growth, and harvest of healthy, naturally grown food. She will provide food as it should be, fresh, no chemicals, grown locally, in season. And it will be the fruits of someone we know and trust. She will restore our connection to the land, Eileen the bridge, bringing us into communion with it. She respects the land, water, sun, and weather, and she knows that working in synchronization with them, she will reap what she sows. (Well, most of the time! She also knows the harvest is *not* in her control, after a certain point.) Someone pouring her own life into working in tandem with the rest of the creation creates new life, new energy, new hope.

Above all, it is hope Eileen bears for us all, the same hope that inspired unknown neighbors to give $80,000 to the venture—hope that life *can* be different from the way we have lived it in this country in the late twentieth century. Hope that food can nourish us rather than sicken us; hope that land can be saved for useful production; hope that the birds and animals and fish that were created to live in bushes and trees and streams will not be driven out of existence by our short-sightedness; hope that the created world will not be completely paved over except for "nature preserves" and parks;

hope that farming the land without chemical pesticides and fertilizers is still a viable way. Through her dedication and perseverance and plenty of plain old determination, Eileen unwittingly became a carrier for the collective, us. An ordinary woman who, with some help, carried off an extraordinary feat, she gave the gift of hope, and in so doing became not just a farmer, but also a healer.

For what is hope if not an agent of healing? Doctors and ministers have long known that hope is necessary to recover health, to grow whole, to survive death-dealing conditions. Hope can carry us through all sorts of awful events, and it can also inspire us in everyday situations. I for one did not know how much I needed Eileen's hope until it blossomed forth. I did not know such deep yearnings were in my soul. Life can be happy, productive, and full, and still something can come along that fills a spot we didn't know was empty, leading to greater wholeness. We know some parts of our lives that need healing, but there are other, lesser known spots in us that need healing too. It is to such places, known or unknown, that hope speaks. Turned, tilled, seeded, watered, hope grows on a suburban farm, there for the harvesting.

· 26 ·

community life

Herman Andrews is ninety-three years old, winning him the title of "Oldest Man in Southampton" at our town's summer gathering, Old Home Days. It's a weekend when people come home from all over to visit with families and friends. Herm would have been awarded the gold cane, given to the oldest *person,* had he not been edged out by Evelyn Kendrick, back visiting relations, age ninety-nine. All he got was a rose!

Herm is a much-beloved man, as was his wife, Dorothy, who died a ways back. Herm lives in his cozy little house, heated by woodstove, though he does have a furnace for backup. Herm still cuts cords and cords of wood, though a lot less than he used to a few years ago when he was still in the business of sugaring. At age ninety, he was up late and rising early to feed the fires for his evaporator, which turns maple sap into syrup. Now he dedicates himself to working his garden, from which he sells produce, including juicy peaches and raspberries, for spending money. Working all day, dawn to dusk, seems to be what keeps Herm going, fit as a fiddle. That, and his faith in God, his obvious and continuing love for his wife, his serene approach to life, and his loving, kind manner with all whom he encounters.

Herm is a model for everyone who is coming up behind him. He shows us what it means to live a good life, a life lived in community, with God and loved ones and neighbor serving as compass points. Herm can generally be found around his home, working in the garden or clearing brush or cutting wood or patching something together. I like to stop by to say hello because he always makes me feel good. He has a special way that makes you feel he is glad to see you. He has lived long enough that not much bothers him about people: that is, he accepts you on your own terms, and you can feel this from him too. He exudes peace, gentleness, and a long view on things. I don't think he is this way simply by virtue of being older: he was always like this, from what I'm told. His wife's death may have opened him up more to people, as sad endings sometimes do. But he has been around long enough to know what's important and what's not, and he acts upon his knowledge, valuing things such as friendship, family, love, generosity, respect, good weather, children singing in church, and an old truck that he can keep running.

As a neighbor, I have had occasion to call on Herm's good graces, and he has helped me out on several occasions. One in particular still makes us laugh together. One day when I was getting dressed, I saw a rat scurry across the floor. I was aghast. We have plenty of mice around here, field mice that come indoors when it starts to get cool, but this was definitely a rat. I slammed the door shut and ran out, hoping it wouldn't slip out somewhere else in the house. I didn't know if I should try to trap it, get someone in to set out poison, or what. That was not long after we had moved to Southampton. I had met Herm in church and liked him a lot, and he seemed to be the type of person I could call on for help. I was pretty sure Herm would have a suggestion. I drove down to his house and found him at home, as he usually is, working. After I told him the problem, he said he'd be up in a few minutes and take care of it.

I returned home and sure enough, Herm was close behind me, but when he got out of his car and came in, he was carrying a rifle! He asked me to lead him to the room, said he was going to shoot the rat there. Herm, said I, I don't want a rat blasted all over the bedroom wall! He said it was a small gauge gun; the rat would remain intact. We went in, waited quietly, Herm with the gun to his chin, and then the rat ran out, toward me. I screamed, throwing off Herm's aim. The rat got away and was never to be seen again. Herm left, disappointed, I think, that he hadn't been able to take his shot; I was relieved, not having been convinced that the rat would die the promised tidy death.

After the rat incident, Herm and I shared something. I think he appreciated being called upon for help, and I appreciated the fact that he didn't repeat the story, as far as I know. Since he has lived so long, he has had ample opportunity to help dozens of people in town in dozens of ways. Over a lifetime of doing such, bonds are formed. Herman, always ready to lend a hand, has many such bonds. Living in community this way, with mutuality at the center, Herm adds to the commonweal by contributing to a greater wholeness for us all, those who live in this place, go to school and church and town meeting together. One such person, weaving threads of connection over a long lifetime lived in the same town, serves the community by how he lives out his life. In Herm's case, the integrity and soundness and kindness that he brings to life act as agents of healing, working in the world to increase the common supply of integrity, soundness, kindness. Positive energy and values loosed into the world heal. Negative energy and lack of values weaken. One older man at work in his garden, living a very ordinary existence, fertilizes the world with what is needed for healthy growth.

a teacher who knows when to come

Ann Belford Ulanov is the Christiane Brooks Johnson Memorial Professor of Psychiatry and Religion at Union Theological Seminary, New York City. Ann's field includes courses on the psychology of prayer, anxiety, identity, fantasy, and religious experience, unusual in terms of the more standard theological and biblical fare offered in most seminaries. Much of the work in building up such a department can be credited to Ann, who teaches at Union, chairs her department, shepherds her students, maintains a private practice of therapy, is a supervising analyst and member of the faculty of the Jung Institute in New York City, writes prolifically (and jointly, with her husband, Barry, McIntosh Professor of English Emeritus at Barnard College and lecturer at Union), mothers her grown children, and manages to take "time off" at a home in Connecticut. A teacher extraordinaire, she imparts what may be more characteristic of a guru than of a distinguished seminary professor, but in fact she is both, and as such, she heals.

Petite, trim, often to be seen with a slight, inquisitive cock to her head, Ann has a knowledge base that is readily apparent and spreads across many fields. The politics of clinical diagnosis, world events, the need for ministers to learn to preach to the soul, the importance of art and poetry to the spirit, biblical dream interpretation, current cinema, the nature of suffering, the latest fashion trend and what it means— all are grist for her mill. Once she has thought them through and reflected upon them, Ann passes processed little nuggets of wisdom along to her students as a mother bird might pass chewed-up bits of worms to her fledglings. This feeding happens in the usual places: lecture hall, seminars, her office. And none of this is so unusual, really, for a professor—we expect a wide range of knowledge (if not necessarily wisdom) from those ensconced in endowed chairs. The distinguishing gift Ann Ulanov possesses is an eye that can see into the soul of anyone who comes before her for long, discerning who that person truly is, what gifts and talents are hers, and where and how she might best use them in the world. A bit of folk wisdom says that someone born with a caul over the head will grow up to have "second sight," the ability to see things others don't. Ann must have been born with a caul.

This seeing Ann does is subtle, certainly not done in secret but not a public kind of activity, either. Her students come to know about it; others might not. It's ordinary in the sense that it can meet you anywhere, but you do have to be open to it to be in a position to receive it. She observes people keenly, using all her senses and intelligences, takes in cues, mixes it all up and stews it, simmering it on a back burner until the time is right. The day then comes when she feeds back to you what she has seen and taken in about you, and it is an astonishing feeling to find yourself so profoundly known by someone who in actuality you barely know! It can have the quality of revelation, so deep, so wise, so knowing it is, what Ann sees. She knows your finest gifts, she apprehends your potentialities, all that you could be, all that lies waiting for you to step into, like a new suit of clothes. All of us live with hidden potential, and we sometimes have glimmerings of it, but because it is nascent and stored in the unconscious, we don't have access to it, can't get hold of it. Ann comes along—there is a saying that when the pupil is ready, the teacher will come, and Ann is the teacher who knows when to come—sizes you up, sees straight into your soul, and then gives you a poke, like a Zen master with a stick (only Ann's tool of choice is the sharpened lance of consciousness). So precise is she in where she pokes that whatever lies waiting emerges. She calls something new into being, and you are never the same.

In my case, among the several nuggets Ann fed back to me about myself over the course of six years, one I remember in particular was this: I went to ask her about a course her husband, Barry, was teaching at Union. It had a class limit, and I wondered if it was still possible to get in. Ann immediately called Barry at home to ask him, and in telling Barry something about me as a student, since he did not know me, said something about my being "original." The experience of hearing that said about me was compelling. It was something I had never considered myself to be, never been called by anyone, and to be so *named* pointed me straight to the source of my creativity, which had been locked off to me since childhood. By identifying a piece of me I was unaware of, Ann gave me permission to claim a dormant part of myself and bring it to life, bring *me* to new life. Ann Ulanov saw me as original? What news! Perhaps I was! What I considered "odd" about myself might be what Ann considered "original. " Being seen through her lens caused something to shift in me. We are apt to name and judge harshly the very parts of ourselves that distinguish us from others, but if someone says, in effect, "Look, this is good, this is rich, this is something you must claim," she makes it easier to stand up to the inner critic. This is a profound kind of support. With that word, she gave me the courage to veer off in new directions, to give voice to what I was thinking (but often left unsaid), to follow my own vision and honor it.

To be so seen, and known, and best of all, affirmed, for *whoever* you are, *whatever* your gifts—such an experience is rare, and precious, and healing. Healing because it calls out parts of yourself that have not had the chance to be known, let alone acted upon, and binds them up in a kind of knitting together of loose pieces. To make contact with unclaimed parts of yourself is healing because it leads to greater whole-ness of being: to be healed *means* to become more whole.

Ann's gift of special sight has much to do with her ability to heal, but another important aspect of that ability is her spa-ciousness of being. She is not filled up with her own ego and agenda. She has "space" that makes her available for such work of the soul. I "got" this about her a while back, driving by a front yard garden that I pass several times a week by car. There used to be a singularly lovely, small, tidy garden in a semicircle toward a front corner. The rest of the yard, not a large one, was simple and green, mostly grass and a few shrubs. The small stand of perennials, chosen carefully for color, height, and season, stood out in spectacular glory against the simplicity of the rest. But then the house was sold, and one spring the new owners were hard at work digging up the yard, adding beds, filling up the previously empty space. By June, one could no longer see anything standing out: it was overloaded, a riot of color, tangled and jarring. It was too much. In this case, less really *was* more. Once it was filled, the beauty of the simple garden was gone.

Like the owner of the first garden, Ann Ulanov maintains a tidy, contained, and well-tended psychic garden, with plenty of spaciousness surrounding it. She can receive people be-cause she is not jammed. We are drawn to anyone who main-tains such fertile space because it gives us a gardenlike place to breathe, to rest, to relax: to be. It offers us an oasis, and when we reach a lush green place with living waters in the midst of the deserts we all traverse, we receive healing of what was dry and parched. As Ezekiel foretold, dry bones can rise up and return to life. Ann gives living water, along with her vision: it's part of who she is. In the far Upper West Side of Manhattan there is healing to be had. This teacher is ready, waiting, for her students. Each of us can be found, seen, healed by our own teacher. We just have to be ready for the teacher, who may be close by to us, waiting.

· 28 ·

no quiet, please!

When I moved to western Massachusetts from Washington, D.C., where I had worked at the Library of Congress for a number of years, one of my lesser fears was that I would not be able to find the books I wanted. I was used to being able to go into the library's stacks (which are closed off now to staff, sad to say, but were open then) and find virtually whatever I wanted. Moving to a town of five thousand people (less than the size of the staff of the library) with a small public library seemed to present a stretch to my reading habits. Ironic, then, and delightedly so, that I would find in Southampton a gem of a library, one that personified the idea of library that readers hold somewhere in their collective memory, library as it was meant to be, soulful and grand and full of vitality.

What makes a library so? The architecture can certainly add to or detract from the archetype. In 1985, when I arrived in town, the library building was a classic red brick, à la Andrew Carnegie, complete with decorative oak moldings and trim work inside. But it was also overflowing, totally out of space, having been designed for a town of less than one thousand people. Books were everywhere. Staff were jammed between piles, with scant space to work in or on. That year the library board launched an initiative for new space: no additions would fit the property lines, and after a protracted effort taking several years, a new building was approved and built adjacent to the town park. It opened two years ago, and now there is plenty of space, a computer center, a room for story hour and crafts next to the children's section, and some five hundred adult new readers, an increase of more than 25 percent, big numbers in library biz. We're all happy and proud of the new library, though it doesn't have the gemütlich quality of the old building. It's not a classic building, but it's certainly adequate.

The quality of the collection is another obvious variable. Ours is, again, quite adequate: strong in some areas, such as gardening, crafts, nature, cookbooks, husbandry, beekeeping (areas relevant to life in this town and therefore very well used), weak in others, with lots of fiction, some good, some so-so.

What makes this particular library an outstanding one, however, is the staff. These librarians keep us all coming, they the lure because they make the library a place where we want to be. I have known many librarians in my day, and this crew, Dorothy and the two Carols, is among the best I've encountered. Because they are who they are, our library is filled with spirit, with fun, with life. We read increasingly of people in the United States feeling the lack of community, leaving cities to move back to Iowa, Wisconsin, South Carolina, wherever they feel they will find a better quality of life, a sense of belonging. But just being outside a city is no guarantee of community: it takes engagement and spirit and effort for a place to become a source of community. And it is just such engagement, spirit, and effort that Dorothy, Carol, and Carol bring to their work at the Edwards Public Library, Southampton, Massachusetts.

Head librarian Dorothy Frary ensures that anyone coming through the door is made to feel welcome. This is not a quiet library—loud greetings are common, followed by laughs, exchange of town news, suggestions of new books that might be of interest. There's always a teenager or two sitting at the desk stamping books under Dorothy's tutelage. She seems to capture young people with ease, and it's clear that they love being there: young people know when someone is authentic and fun, and pays attention to them as real people. Adults, too, are drawn to Dorothy because she knows what's going on and can make us laugh, but also because she is soulful. We can spot it in her eyes, and it's fundamental to who she is, along with her witty take on the world. So she draws us in with her attitude and the atmosphere created, and then delivers the goods. Dorothy is a voracious reader, knows books backward and forward, and knows her clientele's tastes as well. She pays attention, knows what books you are drawn to, holds new ones as special treats. Further, she seems to remember every fact she has ever learned, so is also a walking reference book, an invaluable resource to the kids coming in to do papers and homework. Overhearing her running commentary while helping a patron is a treat in itself: facts mixed with Dorothy's take on the facts, delivered with the aplomb of a professional comedian and generally hilarious.

Carol Goulet is the library technician who does processing and, of particular interest to me, orders books on interlibrary loan. She works most often in the back, often at the computer, but her presence is nonetheless vividly felt because she anchors the place with a sense of order. Gentle, modest, the quietest of the three, Carol soothes and calms with her patient approach to life. Her welcome conveys her readiness to assist you in finding what you need: she's willing. With me, it's those interlibrary loans. I come with snippets torn out of the *New York Times Book Review* or jottings that I've made while reading, incomplete citations, scrawled in writing I can't read. Carol patiently scrolls through the computer files until she finds a match. It's extra work in a busy place, but she never acts put out or hurried. She works at her own pace, and that pace envelops whomever she is with. She extends herself generously, and the spirit of her generosity emanates from her perch behind the glass panels.

Carol Freebourn is the free spirit who runs the children's section. She reigns over a queendom of delight, installed as she is among puppets, toys, cardboard houses to crawl into, tiny tea sets, and books, books, books! Carol is an old hand at her work—she has been at it for some years—but to each child she brings fresh delight and attention, as if he or she were the first and only child to walk into the room that day. Given to colorful jewelry and clothes, Carol is an enchantress, weaving her tales and spinning her thread around every child, making him or her into a reader. She is fun; the library is fun; reading is fun! A simple and elegant approach that works, this making of reading into a delight. (She had 330 children enrolled in the last summer reading program, for example, of which 225 completed the assignment of reading six books.) It works because of who *she is*. She is alive, passionate about this work of getting children to love books, to read. A genuine engagement she has with children, it is more than a job; it is a calling. With her enchanted calling, Carol the fairy godmother taps with her wand, bringing to her charges a gift that will nourish them through a lifetime, the gift of story, the gift of reading, the gift of a librarian they will remember, because she extended herself to them with such zest.

This library isn't really about books, though books are its mission. It's about people. People, older and younger and in-between, wanting to be seen for who they are. People wanting to belong in this world, to have at least one place in the community they can go to and be assured they are both known and welcomed.

Dorothy, Carol, and Carol, in bringing the full force of their lively selves to bear upon the library, create such a place.

Not the building, not the books, but the spirit of life is what Southampton's library is about. No musty repository of knowledge here; rather, life in full swing, loud, vibrant, playful, full of raucous laughter and fun, sometimes silly, occasionally quiet, but never, ever dull, it gives life, and so heals. You must take from the life source wherever and whenever it bubbles up. A small public library might not be where you would ordinarily think to go to be infused with life's energy, but that's what's extraordinary! Find a moment of healing in such an ordinary place.

minister's minister

Lee Hancock is a minister's minister, and there is none finer. She is the minister people long for, and she delivers what they need: love, understanding, wisdom, wit, and witness, all informed, and formed, by her deeply rooted and broadly embracing faith. All this, and the gift of healing, placed in the service of a God more expansive than many of us know. Because of her bigness, her widely inclusive spirit, her huge, compassionate heart, Lee is able to minister more broadly and deeply than most, and she moves through the world touching lives in much the way Jesus did—and appealing to the same sorts of people.

Mother of two adolescent daughters, Hannah and Sarah, wife of Mark, a producer, faithful daughter-in-law to Mark's mother, Sue, who lives with them, and colleague and friend to hundreds, Lee has the capacity to know, help, and keep up with more people, and immerse herself in more projects, than anyone I have ever met. Trench coat flapping, bag overstuffed, needing to make a quick call home, Lee is a study in perpetual motion, which makes it all the more amazing that when she stops, settles, and is with you, she can push all this aside in her mind, focus, be entirely present, and make you feel that you are precisely the person she has been wanting to see!

Lee has rheumatoid arthritis, which has left its mark on her: it slows her walk at times, although she generally moves along at a pretty fast clip. You can spot Lee coming from a distance and know it is she. She looks around while moving along, swiveling her head back and forth, observing and taking in whatever is there. She doesn't miss a trick, functioning like a radar screen, with particular sensitivities to people and their energies, moods, states of mind. Her ability to take in, sort, intuit, and interpret in the midst of all that she has going on is nothing short of amazing, for Lee always has things cooking in her life, much, much more than seems humanly possible.

Recently, for instance, Lee has been involved in serving persons with AIDS in Newark, New Jersey, where she is responsible for the program office of the Newark Project, an effort combining urban ministry, advocacy, and ethnography. She teaches religion as an adjunct instructor at Drew Theological School (from which she will receive her Ph.D.), is a pastoral associate at a church in New York where she conducts a monthly healing service, is considering a run for her local school board, is involved in writing a proposal for a mammoth grant for the Newark Project, is editing a book of sermons by women preachers that is due at her publisher as soon as possible, and is writing her dissertation on suffering (specifically, why some people's lives are transformed by suffering, and others' destroyed), a subject she knows all too well. Lee constructed the idea of "witnessing to suffering" as a dissertation subject, and in discussing it with her some time ago, I saw that indeed that is what Lee does, who she is: a witness to suffering.

Full of life and spirit, Lee is also great fun to be with, often arrives for a visit with a good champagne (which she drinks with zeal), always with a screamingly funny story or two to tell, as well as exciting new intellectual and theological pursuits. She is generous to a fault, most notably with her time, which is why she is sometimes behind schedule. Not infrequently needing a last-minute favor from someone to help her out of a "squeeze play," Lee is afforded more grace by her friends and colleagues than anyone I know, and with good reason. People who have ever made a connection with Lee know that when push comes to shove, she will be there for them, present and ready to witness whatever needs witnessing, whether that is dying a tortured death or providing a thoughtful analysis of a particular situation. Because she knows how to witness, and chooses to do so, she heals.

The "job" of witnessing to human suffering is the role of the minister, or should be. It is one of the toughest jobs a person can do, and many people probably would not pursue ordination if they really knew what was going to be required of them. But they *cannot* know about it until immersed in it for a measure of time. And there are those who, realizing what they have gotten into, choose to wall themselves off from the daily dose of pain, understandably so, because unless one has done the necessary work of learning to know, support, and nourish oneself along the way, one could soon sink under the burden. Ministers are notoriously bad at caring for themselves, and anyone who cannot care for himself or herself cannot care for another human being. Compassion begins with compassion for our own pain, our own suffering. We cannot extend to another what we do not have within ourselves.

Lee is able to witness to suffering because she has endured her own and transformed it into a capacity for healing what ails others. That, and because she is *willing* to take on the job, a rare decision. People such as Lee are indeed called to their work by God, but God gets few responses, from what I've seen. "Many are called but few are chosen" explains that those called to labor for God may decline the offer (and usually do). Scarce are the people who are willing to voluntarily be present to those who suffer. When the choice is made to do so, there is no turning back, because once acquainted with the enormity and varieties of human suffering, the one called will always know it's there, inescapable. Suffering cannot be avoided once one has knowledge of it. For that reason the young prince Gautama Buddha's father tried to shield him from suffering by never letting him go beyond the palace walls. To say yes to the role of witness is at the same time to say no to any naiveté left lurking in one's soul. The witness necessarily comes to know the dark side, the song of innocence replaced by the song of experience. Nevertheless, someone must do it, and Lee was called, said yes, and nonetheless manages to walk lightly on this earth, a Johnny Appleseed of the spirit, seeding new life wherever she goes.

What does it mean to witness? It is a way of being entirely present with someone, conveying to the sufferer that he or she is not alone in the pain, and that the anguish he or she may be undergoing is not meaningless. Lee does this, in part, by meeting the person as an equal. There is no whiff of pity about her, just the placing of herself so that she can "stand with." Not assuage, not make better (she knows she may not be able to), not do any of the little tricks most of us resort to when we are confronted by a person in pain. She witnesses by *not* doing just as much as by doing, and by backing away enough so that there is room for God to be at work. How many times I have heard her say she needs to "make space for grace!" It's true. She does that because she knows she *can't* do anything on her own, most likely, but can do everything, or at least something, when she relies on God to enter in. Such a practice takes enormous restraint. We want so much to jump in, to give advice, to fix. From amidst the whirlwind of her energy, Lee centers in, she focuses, she listens, she nods, she affirms and supports, and she rocks in her rocking chair, setting up a rhythm that slows the pace. Then quiet can come, and calm, and a measure of relief.

To come to such a point of stillness, of not-doing, takes enormous confidence and enormous faith that God will indeed be present. When it happens, this coming together with God, the moment expands; it is, in fact, outside time, and it is a healing moment. The sufferer has been seen, heard, and understood. The sufferer knows he or she is no longer alone. The sufferer has experienced the love of God through this remarkable, yet also ordinary, person, Lee, who has consented to take on such extraordinary tasks, and yet still lives in the world of overdue school papers, cupcakes for a daughter's class, runaway dogs, husband away on a business trip, all the details of life often persuading us that is all there *is* to life.

But there *is* more, and there *are* ways to be healed, and they are available around us, in suburban houses, in schools, in churches. Lee Hancock lives in those places and shows it is so. She heals through who she is, by what she has experienced, by all she knows, all of which she is able to marshal into whatever time she has to give a person and concentrate it into a dose of love. Received, it is capable of galvanizing a healing response. Totally concentrated loving energy: available to Lee from God, and her own, the force of which carries new life to what ails.

afterword

It's a risky business to use the word "healing." I am aware of all that is stirred up by the very word, especially when used in a religious context. If healing comes from God, why wouldn't God grant it to everyone? Surely a loving God who desires our wholeness wants us to be healthy? And if someone is faithful and true and loving and good, but not healed, what does that say about his or her relationship with God? I get questions along these lines that I can't answer because I don't know the answer, nor will I ever.

I don't know why healing *doesn't* happen. I just know that it can and does. Sometimes healing is manifested in the body, and sometimes in the soul. I know more about soul healing because that's what I deal with much more often as a minister—that is what I feel I was called to do by God: help souls heal themselves.

Every single person who walks this earth needs healing, whether she or he knows it or not. We grow toward wholeness over a lifetime, each of us starting out with certain capacities, lacking others. A human being can move toward wholeness only with the help of other human beings and the help of God. To move toward wholeness is what I call healing; another piece of yourself, no matter how small, is filled in, and you are that much closer to being the person you have the inherent potential to be. And as we move through life, we are wounded along the way, so while some bits of us are in the process of emerging more fully, others get hurt, become pockets of pain small or large, create tears in the fabric of our lives and need healing too. The cycle goes on continually throughout a lifetime.

In a constant process of balancing, we are at any one moment more whole or less so. As we become more conscious of this process, as recesses of pain emerge, disenfranchised parts of ourselves cry out for attention, and if we trust ourselves enough to listen to what we need, then we can begin to open to the agents of healing that are always around us. I have tried to write about some of these agents because it is crucial to know that help does exist, and in fact surrounds us at all times, if we can learn to see it and open to it.

Life itself carries healing for us. We are created that way, so that we can be healed by the very life we are embedded in. How else could it come? Nature, beauty, quiet, proportion— these are aspects of life that can be had by most of us, with a little seeking perhaps, but there for the taking. And there are the healing qualities of people, from whom we can receive such great benefit. The qualities I have named in these stories, and many more, are also part of the life in which we are all embedded—attentiveness, focus, generosity of spirit, trust, inclusivity, respect, compassion, witness, hope, mercy, empathy. Such qualities were given us by God as part of who we are, or can be, "ordinary" qualities with which human beings are endowed, becoming extraordinary when they grow so strong in a person that they can be felt immediately in his or her presence. When someone has come to a point of being completely his or her self, with no masks, no barriers, so that any special qualities can shine clearly through, then presence itself can be healing, and powerfully so.

What this says, in the end, is that we are indeed beings who need each other, and the more fully we can recognize and live into that need, the more whole we will become. We can experience wholeness in the here and now if we open to each other's best qualities, giving and receiving of all God has endowed us with, all that has been given to each of us to use and share.

Growing into wholeness is a mutual enterprise. We cannot do it on our own. We need each other's healing gifts, and conversely, our gifts need to be received for us to be able to share them. And, of course, it is a mutual enterprise with God, with us opening and responding to all the great gifts of healing with which God is ready to grace us.

The people I have named in this book share one thing in common: they are, in whatever way they might express it, aware of their place in the web of mutuality that is life. Each person has a gift and knows it is his or hers to share. To a greater or lesser extent, each one creates his or her life around the sharing of that gift, for it is the thing that gives meaning to life. Money, status, power, and possessions mean little to them, as far as I can tell. What is significant is the opportunity to be an agent in this world, an agent of something bigger and more significant than they would be otherwise.

Being an agent can be an exacting job, for it can take everything a person has and more. I have not written about people who are trying to "do good." I have written about people who are willing to pay a sometimes significant price in order to live according to what is most essential and true for *their* lives. They have given themselves to something that benefits us all: they carry something for the human community. They are our friends, our teachers, our neighbors. They are our healers. To God is the glory, but to them should go our thanks. Here is mine: thank you, dear people, for sharing your considerable gifts, for making the choices you have made, for sharing your selves so generously with the world. And thank you, too, for letting me write about you. It has been pure pleasure!